CLINICAL FOCUS SERIES

Lesions of Sarcoidosis

A Problem Solving Approach

CLINICAL FOCUS SERIES

Lesions of Sarcoidosis

A Problem Solving Approach

Editors

Late Om P Sharma MD FRCP Master FCCP

Violeta Mihailovic-Vucinic MD PhD
Professor of Internal Medicine and Pulmonology
Medical Faculty, University of Belgrade, Serbia
Head of Department of Sarcoidosis and Other Granulomatous Diseases
Clinic of Pulmonology, Clinical Center Belgrade, Serbia
Founder of the Serbian Association of Sarcoidosis

Foreword

Robert P Baughman
Elyse E Lower

JAYPEE

JAYPEE BROTHERS MEDICAL PUBLISHERS (P) LTD.

New Delhi • London • Philadelphia • Panama

Jaypee Brothers Medical Publishers (P) Ltd

Headquarters

Jaypee Brothers Medical Publishers (P) Ltd
4838/24, Ansari Road, Daryaganj
New Delhi 110 002, India
Phone: +91-11-43574357
Fax: +91-11-43574314
Email: jaypee@jaypeebrothers.com

Overseas Offices

J.P. Medical Ltd
83 Victoria Street, London
SW1H 0HW (UK)
Phone: +44-2031708910
Fax: +02-03-0086180
Email: info@jpmedpub.com

Jaypee Medical Inc
The Bourse
111 South Independence Mall East
Suite 835, Philadelphia, PA 19106, USA
Phone: +1 267-519-9789
Email: joe.rusko@jaypeebrothers.com

Jaypee Brothers Medical Publishers (P) Ltd
Bhotahity, Kathmandu, Nepal
Phone: +977-9741283608
Email: Kathmandu@jaypeebrothers.com

Jaypee-Highlights Medical Publishers Inc
City of Knowledge, Bld. 237, Clayton
Panama City, Panama
Phone: +1 507-301-0496
Fax: +1 507-301-0499
Email: cservice@jphmedical.com

Jaypee Brothers Medical Publishers (P) Ltd
17/1-B Babar Road, Block-B, Shaymali
Mohammadpur, Dhaka-1207
Bangladesh
Mobile: +08801912003485
Email: jaypeedhaka@gmail.com

Website: www.jaypeebrothers.com
Website: www.jaypeedigital.com

Inquiries for bulk sales may be solicited at: jaypee@jaypeebrothers.com

Lesions of Sarcoidosis: A Problem Solving Approach

First Edition: **2014**

ISBN 978-93-5090-423-7

Printed at: Samrat Offset Pvt. Ltd.

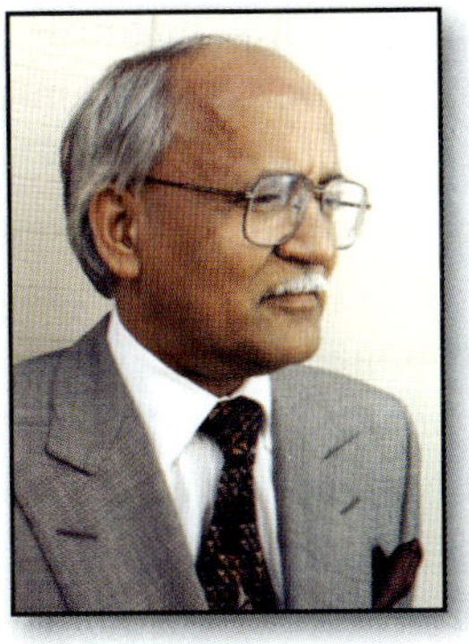

Dedication

Professor Om P Sharma (1936-2012) was born in India, graduated from Victoria College, and attended G.R. Medical College—both in his native land. He then studied tropical medicine at the London School of Hygiene and Tropical Medicine. He served internships in medicine in India, Scotland, and England and a residency at Albert Einstein Medical College, Bronx, New York, where he also completed the fellowship in cardiopulmonary medicine.

Dr Sharma was Professor of Medicine at the Keck School of Medicine at the University of Southern California, Los Angeles, for over 40 years. Dr Sharma was also Professor of Medicine in Residence at Kyoto University Medical School, Kyoto, Japan, 1987-88. He was emeritus President of the World Association of Sarcoidosis and other Granulomatous Disorders (WASOG) and Editor of *Current Opinion in Pulmonary Medicine*.

During his lifetime, Professor Sharma authored or edited eight books, two medical biographies, eight monographs, and has written over 500 articles, short papers, editorials and reviews on the topics of sarcoidosis, tropical medicine, hypersensitivity pneumonitis, interstitial lung disease, other pulmonary disorders, as well as the history of medicine.

This is the last book Professor Sharma wrote. His original idea for the book, Lesions of Sarcoidosis: Problem Solving Approach rose in the summer of 2011. Although suffering with a devastating disease, he had brilliant ideas about how this book should look and how it would contribute both to doctors and patients.

His list of chapters was outstanding but demanding, as was always his scientific approach.

"There are many lesions of sarcoidosis", Professor Sharma wrote in discussing this book with me, and how he imagined our whole project from cover to cover: "We need to make a list of these lesions and then write a chapter on each. Each chapter should be not large; it should be easily readable, contain nice image(s) of the lesion (one, maybe two), a table of differential diagnosis, and brief clinical importance. I envision this book as a clinical book for trainees, general practitioners, and internists.... Of course it will be useful to specialists as well."

Enthusiasm, an endless enthusiasm, is the only way to describe his work on this book—chapter upon chapter, piles of text with such an ease and simplicity. Professor Sharma was an exceptional writer.

"Variety is a spice of life", he used to say, trying to find different cases for each chapter. None are similar to the previous ones. "Sarcoidosis has many faces..."

Professor Sharma wrote while on chemotherapy, he wrote from the bed recovering, he wrote from everywhere. Unfortunately, he did not manage to see this book published, although it was almost finished a couple of weeks before his death.

"In nothing do men more nearly approach the gods than in giving health to men..." These ever inspiring words of Cicero accurately represent the entire life path and the dedication of Professor Sharma whose driving purpose was to give health to his patients.

This book, the last one, is only a small contribution to his life's work.

Violeta Mihailovic-Vucinic

Contents

Preface

Sarcoidosis is a multisystem granulomatous disease of unknown cause and unpredictable course. Since the first description of the mysterious skin lesions of Lady Mortimer by Jonathan Hutchinson, more than one century ago, sarcoidosis remains a puzzling disease in many aspects. Although remarkable advances in investigations of etiology, pathogenesis, and management of sarcoidosis have been made, it still remains inexplicable in many clinical points.

The book "Lesions of Sarcoidosis: A Problem Solving Approach" is the last one written by Professor Sharma. His original idea was that this book would be of use not only to pulmonologists and internists, but also for practitioners of other specialists because of multisystem nature of sarcoidosis.

Professor Sharma sincerely hoped that this book should be a picturesque guide for all doctors who ever intended to explore numerous manifestations of this mysterious disease.

The main purpose of the book is to provide medical fraternity a comprehensive review of possible clinical presentations of sarcoidosis.

Unfortunately, Professor Sharma did not manage to see the book finally published, although he spent his last days busy working on it. Working on this book with him, I was truly amazed with his enormous energy and enthusiasm he enriched each single chapter with.

Writing this preface instead of Professor Sharma is heartbreaking and hard task.

I try to remember how he envisioned the whole book; at the same time I try not to forget all the persons who contributed in each conceivable way to the final look of this book as certainly he would do.

The book "Lesions of Sarcoidosis" was supported by our sarcoidosis patients as Professor Sharma used to say: "who are permanently teaching us about many faces of this mysterious disease".

The support of our families was of the utmost value: Margaret Sharma who helped with all her heart in all necessary details about the final look of this book; my sons Dr Nikola Vucinic and Strahinja-Laza, were supporting me in all difficult moments.

I am particularly grateful to the whole medical staff of the Vth Clinical Department-Clinic of Pulmonary Diseases, University Clinical Center Belgrade, who helped me with this work. My appreciations to the efforts of my Chief of Staff—the

Main Nurse of the Vth Clinical Department, Mrs Ruzica Nikodijevic on helping me in every possible way.

Kind appreciations to my dear colleagues Professor Elyse E Lower and Professor Robert P Baughman from the University of Cincinnati for the breathtaking foreword.

The final look of this book was made by painstaking efforts of Dr Madhu Choudhary, Senior Editor Jaypee Brothers Medical Publishers team and my most sincere appreciations belongs to her.

Authors appreciate all sarcoidosis patients from every conceivable corner of the world for their assistance. They are permanently teaching us about many faces of this mysterious disease.

Violeta Mihailovic-Vucinic

Foreword

Robert P Baughman MD
Professor of Medicine, Department of Medicine
University of Cincinnati Medical Center, Cincinnati, OH, USA

Elyse E Lower MD
Professor of Medicine, Department of Medicine
University of Cincinnati Medical Center, Cincinnati, OH, USA

Professor Jacques Chretien once said: "If you have seen five cases of sarcoidosis, you know nothing about sarcoidosis. If you have seen 50 cases of sarcoidosis, you know everything about sarcoidosis. If you have seen 500 cases of sarcoidosis, you know nothing about sarcoidosis." For many clinicians, sarcoidosis remains an elusive disease without a clear-cut etiology and no specific test which confirms the diagnosis in all cases. Although the disease can affect virtually all organ systems, there is no area of the body, including the lung, which is always involved. Additionally, radiographic and blood tests frequently fail to correlate with clinical symptoms. Some patients will be asymptomatic but display markedly abnormal chest X-rays; whereas, other patients may suffer from extreme cough, dyspnea, and fatigue but have normal chest imaging.

The multiorgan nature of sarcoidosis can both be a blessing and a curse. The finding of granulomas in two or more organs can be a blessing for confirming the diagnosis of sarcoidosis. Because the combination of eye and lung disease supports the diagnosis of sarcoidosis, a patient with mediastinal adenopathy and active uveitis is more likely to have sarcoidosis and less likely to have Hodgkin's lymphoma. However, this multisystem involvement may also be a curse when a patient presents to a neurologist or cardiologist who infrequently treats sarcoidosis and hence fails to recognize this granulomatous process.

"Lessons of sarcoidosis" provides a unique approach to assist clinicians in better understanding the multifaceted nature of this disease. In contrast to most standard textbooks which summarize tables and figures for the "average" sarcoidosis patient, Professors Sharma and Mihailovic-Vucinic have provided clinical scenarios that may be encountered by practicing clinicians faced with diagnosing and treating sarcoidosis. This practical venue enables the clinician to appreciate the vast differences in patient presentation, organ involvement, and outcomes seen in sarcoidosis. Clinical vignettes examine both focused questions important for some specific patients, such as lupus pernio, as well as more generalized issues common to most sarcoidosis patients, such as pain, dyspnea, and fatigue.

The prestigious authors of this book have successfully managed thousands of patients from two international sarcoidosis clinics for many years. Because of this extensive combined expertise, this book reflects a shared international experience for both the usual and the unusual aspects of the disease.

We believe that after reading this book one will be not only as enthralled with sarcoidosis as we are but also have a better understanding of this chameleon like disease.

CHAPTER

1 Sarcoidosis: A Worldwide Disease

INTRODUCTION

Sarcoidosis is an illness that generates tremendous anxiety amongst those who suffer from it and creates academic interest amongst those who provide care to the sufferers. The disease occurs throughout the world and has been with us for more than 150 years.

HISTORICAL ACCOUNT

In 1869, Jonathan Hutchinson, a British dermatologist described a 58-year-old coal-wharf worker with purple symmetrical skin plaques on the legs and hands that had gradually developed over the preceding 2 years. The lesions were neither tender nor painful. The patient also had suffered from gout and finally died of renal failure. This most likely was the first case of clinically described sarcoidosis. In the earlier decades of the 20th century, sarcoidosis was not a significant illness; its evidence remained surrounded in the veil of tuberculosis.[1-3]

In 1936, the first significant publication about sarcoidosis appeared in America; it was a 75-page review from Johns Hopkins Hospital by Warfield Longcope. This event took place almost 6 decades after the first recorded case of sarcoidosis by Hutchinson.[4] The first epidemiological study on sarcoidosis appeared in 1950, based on 350 cases detected in World War II US veterans. In army inductees, the rates in African-Americans and Caucasians were 17.8 and 0.9, respectively, in 350 cases; whereas, in 134 African-Americans and Caucasians Navy recruits, the rates of sarcoidosis were 81.8 and 7.6, respectively. The most recent data from enlisted navy men shows an annual incidence rate of 16.0 for African-Americans and 2.5 for Caucasians.[5]

Scadding defined sarcoidosis as a disease characterized by the formation in all of several affected tissues of epithelioid-cell tubercles without caseation, though fibrinoid necrosis may be present at the center of a few, proceeding either to resolution or to conversion into hyaline fibrous tissue. This definition emphasizes only the histological features of the illness. The knowledge of the disease is vast now and that we need to include not only the clinical, but also the radiological, immunological, biochemical, and the genetic aspects of the illness. Sarcoidosis, a multisystem disorder of unknown cause, commonly affects young and middle-aged adults, and frequently presents with bilateral hilar adenopathy, pulmonary infiltration, ocular, and skin lesions. The liver, spleen, lymph nodes, salivary glands, heart, nervous system, muscles, bones, and other organs may also be involved. The diagnosis is established when clinicoradiographic findings are supported by histological evidence of noncaseating epithelioid cell granulomas. Granulomas of unknown causes and local sarcoid reactions must be excluded. Frequently observed immunological features are depression of cutaneous delayed type-hypersensitivity and a heightened T helper cell 1 immune response at sites of disease. Circulating immune-complexes along with signs of β-cell hyperactivity may also be found.[6]

In 1974, Louis Siltzbach in a world review, "Course and Prognosis of Sarcoidosis", published in the *Am J Med.*, emphasized that there was an extraordinary parallelism in prognosis of sarcoidosis in different ethnic groups, living in radically different environments and climates. If the patient presented with hilar adenopathy, resolution was to be expected without any treatment; but if lung infiltrates were present, resolution was less likely even with steroid therapy. Depending on the period of observation, the mortality due to sarcoidosis was less than 5%.[7]

In 2001, a case control etiologic study of sarcoidosis (ACCESS), conducted by Baughman et al., finally established the clinical epidemiological features in 736 patients, 53% white and 44% black, with sarcoidosis from 10 clinical centers in the US. There were more females than males who were more likely to have eye lesions, neurological involvement, and erythema nodosum, whereas men were likely to have hypercalcemia. Black patients were more likely to have chronic skin lesions and eye, liver, bone marrow, and lymph node involvement. The organ involvement depended on the race, age, and sex of the patient. The exploration of environmental and occupational factors did not reveal a single predominant cause of sarcoidosis. Insecticides, agricultural environments, and bioaerosols exposures were associated with sarcoidosis.[8]

The disease occurs worldwide. Its frequency, pulmonary and extrapulmonary manifestations, response to treatment, and prognosis are extraordinarily similar. Furthermore, there are certain distinctive features of the disease related to geography and race. This book provides a plan to recognize and manage the common and less common lesions of sarcoidosis (Figure 1-1).

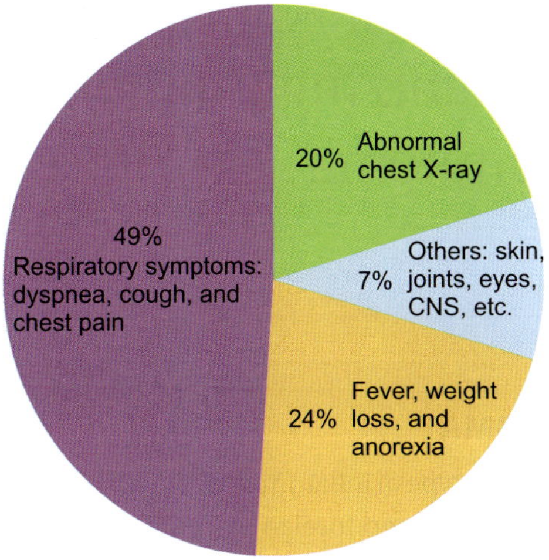

Figure 1-1 Presenting features of multisystem sarcoidosis. CNS, central nervous system. *Source:* Sharma OP. Sarcoidosis: Clinical Management. London: Butterworths; 1984. p. 23.

REFERENCE

1. Hutchinson J. Anomalous diseases of skin and fingers: case of livid papillary psoriasis? In: Hutchinson J, editor. Illustrations of Clinical Surgery. London: J and A Churchill; 1877. p. 42-3.
2. Hutchinson J. Mortimer's malady: a form of lupus pernio. *Arch Surg (London).* 1898;9:307-15.
3. Hunter FT. Hutchinson-Boeck's disease (generalized sarcoidosis): historical note and report of a case with apparent cure. *New Engl J Med.* 1936;214:246-52.
4. Longcope W. The generalized form of Boeck's sarcoid. *Trans Assoc Am Physicians.* 1936;51;94-102.
5. Gupta D, Sharma OP. Sarcoidosis. In: Jindal SK editor. Textbook of pulmonary and critical care disease. New Delhi: Jaypee Brothers Medical Publishers; 2011. p. 1188-216.
6. Scadding JG, Mitchell D. Sarcoidosis. 2nd ed. London: Chapman and Hall; 1985.
7. James DG. Sarcoidosis and respiratory disorders: Festschrift in honour of Louis Siltzbach. *Mt Sinai J Med.* 1977;44:683-879.
8. Baughman RP, Teirstein AS, Judson MA, Rossman MD, Yeager H Jr, Bresnitz EA, et al. Clinical characteristics of patients in a case control study of sarcoidosis. *Am J Respir Crit Care Med.* 2001;164:1885-9.

CHAPTER 2 A Clinical Approach to Recognizing Pulmonary Granulomas

WHAT IS GRANULOMA?

Granuloma is a nonspecific type of inflammatory response which may be triggered by various antigenic agents or by inert foreign materials. The antigens cause activation of the cellular immune system—lymphocytes and macrophages. Granulomas are formed as the result of the complex interaction of cytokines produced by these cells. The antigenic triggering agents include a wide variety of infectious agents (mycobacteria, fungi, etc.), beryllium, the unknown antigen(s), responsible for sarcoidosis, and numerous other antigens.[1] Foreign bodies induced granulomas are commonly considered to be nonimmunologic in origin.

Granulomatous reaction may be classified functionally into 2 major categories.[1] The first group consists of lesions characterized by delayed-type hypersensitivity, antigen specific response. These granulomas are very active lesions with a pretty high rate of cell turnover. The granulomas of delayed-type hypersensitivity are seen in tuberculosis (TB), sarcoidosis, hypersensitivity pneumonitis, and schistosomiasis. The second type is foreign body granulomas that lack an antigen specific response. These types of granulomas are often inactive lesions with minimal destruction and quite low cell turnover. The granulomas of the second type are seen in berylliosis, where the agent causing granulomas is inert.

CAUSES OF GRANULOMAS

There are numerous causes of granulomatous diseases. The causes vary from live, replicating intracellular organisms, such as bacteria, mycobacteria, virus, or fungi to metazoans (helminthes), substances like metals or chemical agents and organic antigens.

Granulomas occur in a variety of respiratory diseases and diseases affecting many other organs. Diffuse granulomatous pulmonary diseases form a heterogeneous group with a variety of clinical presentations.[2,3]

In the following text, granulomatous diseases affecting lungs are summarized and for easier understanding divided into 2 main groups: infectious and non-infectious.

DIAGNOSTIC APPROACH

Infectious Granulomatous Diseases

Infectious granulomatous diseases are important group of granulomatous disorders and the differential diagnoses is mandatory considering their prevalence, clinical heterogeneity, and the available therapeutic possibilities. The initial approach usually includes a search for the alcohol-acid-resistant bacillus (Ziehl-Neelsen staining) and mycobacteria detection, and silver-methenamine staining (Grocott staining) to identify fungi.[4-6] Nocardia can also be detected by these methods. It is estimated that 106 microorganisms per millimeter of tissue are required for Ziehl-Neelsen staining to be positive.[6]

If there is a clinical-radiological suspicion, a search for bronchocentric granulomatosis antigen can be performed for mycobacteria, and for fungus antigens of *Pneumocystis brasiliensis* and *Pneumocystis carinii*. Polymerase chain reaction (PCR) can be used in histological pictures suspected of mycobacteriosis, where the infectious agent was not identified by other methods.[6,7] A positive PCR result is not considered valid from the diagnostic viewpoint unless one or more microorganisms can be identified inside the tissue by the Ziehl-Neelsen technique. Recently, QuantiFERON-TB Gold test is broadly appreciated.

If this group of reactions was unable to identify an infectious agent, the histological and radiological characteristics are fundamental for the clinical management and establishment of possible diagnosis while waiting for the microbiological culture result.[8]

Noninfectious Granulomatous Diseases

Each noninfectious granulomatous pulmonary disease represents unique clinical and radiological characteristics. However, these characteristics may present various degrees of overlapping. The differences reflected by the histological presentation of each disease allow differential diagnosis with a certain degree of precision.

CLINICAL APPROACH TO DIFFERENTIAL DIAGNOSIS OF MYCOBACTERIAL GRANULOMATOUS DISEASES

Mycobacterial Infections: Tuberculosis

Despite the medical achievements of the 21st century, TB remains the leading cause of illness and death from infectious diseases all over the world. Tropical countries, especially, bear the brunt of the global TB burden.[1,9] TB is a multisystem granulomatous disorder, so patients should be examined for different organs involvement (skin, eye, and peripheral lymph nodes).

Clinical Presentation

Typical evening rise of temperature may also indicate TB infection. Unilateral hilar adenopathy (as in primary TB), miliary infiltrates, or upper lobes infiltrates with or without cavity are characteristics of this infection.

Tuberculin skin test (Figure 2-1) may have a certain role to support the diagnosis, however, the test cannot distinguish latent infection from active disease.

Bacillus Calmette-Guérin (BCG) vaccination which is widely administered in many countries with high incidence of TB infection also results in positive tuberculin skin tests that persist in adults.[10] Elevated serum angiotensin converting enzyme (ACE) levels and hypercalcemia may occur in miliary TB but it is not of significance for definite diagnosis.

Generally, TB does not cause eosinophilia. A typical undulating blood eosinophilia may correlate with disease activity. High count of eosinophils in patients with pulmonary TB usually indicates an improvement.[11] The radiological features of TB are described in figure 2-2.

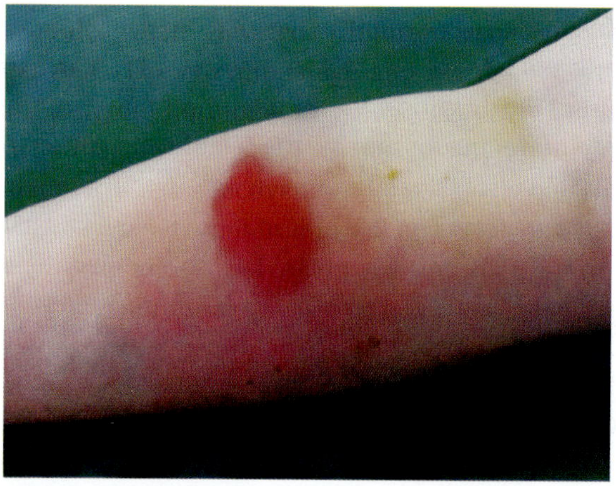

Figure 2-1 Positive tuberculin skin test in a patient with active tuberculosis.

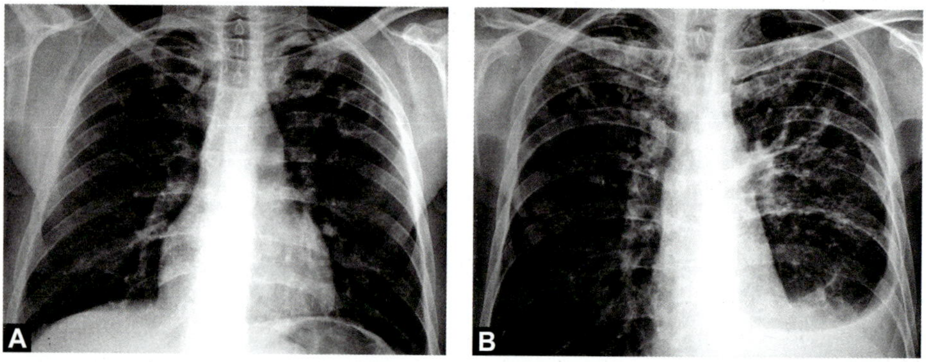

Figure 2-2 Radiological features of tuberculosis may broadly vary; however, in a majority of patients, tuberculosis is presented with **A,** cavitary lesions localized in the upper lobes of the lungs and sometimes **B,** the lesions are accompanied by pleural effusion of the same side.

Mycobacterial Infections: Nontuberculosis

Approximately 100 species, characterized by the lipid-rich cell walls compose the *Mycobacterium* genus. The general characteristic is acid-fast staining. The *Mycobacterium* genus contains 2 obligate pathogens: the *Mycobacterium tuberculosis* complex (*M. bovis, M. africanum, M. microfti,* and *M. canetti*) and *Mycobacterium leprae.*

Other species of the *Mycobacterium* genus live freely in the environment and are called "environment mycobacteria (EM)" or non-TB mycobacteria. Some species of EM cause opportunistic infections in humans (*M. avium* complex and *M. kansasii*).

Clinical Presentation

Most patients are men with history of smoking, chronic obstructive pulmonary disease, bronchiectasis, rheumatoid lung, healed TB lesions, exposure to dust with underlying lung damage as pneumoconiosis, or silicosis.[12,13]

Pulmonary disease due to EM occurs as a component of disseminated infection but often the disease affects only lungs. The major problem in definite diagnosis of pulmonary disease caused by EM is the establishment of clinical significance of these organisms isolated from sputum and other pulmonary specimens by culture or by acid stain based techniques.[14]

Leprosy

Leprosy is still one of the most important infectious diseases that affects millions of people worldwide. *M. leprae,* the cause of the disease is highly infective but low in pathogenicity, with the preference to grow in cool parts of the body.

Clinical Presentation

The clinical presentation of leprosy generally depends on the host immune response to the infections. In lepromatous leprosy (LL), the cellular immune response is not activated. The disease is characterized by widespread skin lesions, erythematous or brown, and papular or nodular eruptions (Figure 2-3). The lesions are not anesthetic. *M. leprae* can be isolated from nasal smears or biopsy specimen taken from intact skin. With the disease progression, the skin becomes thickened producing typical leonine face. The lepromin test is usually negative in LL and positive in tuberculoid leprosy (TL). ACE levels may be increased in leprosy.

Patients with TL have more effective cellular immune response. These patients are presented with the serious damage of the peripheral nerves mediated by delayed type hypersensitivity reactions to mycobacterial antigen located in sheaths and fibers. There is a certain nerve predilection: the ulnar, median, radial, lateral popliteal, and greater auricular. This neuropathy leads to specific palsies. The anesthesia leads to ulcerations and loss of tissue. The granulomas have little or no caseation, and

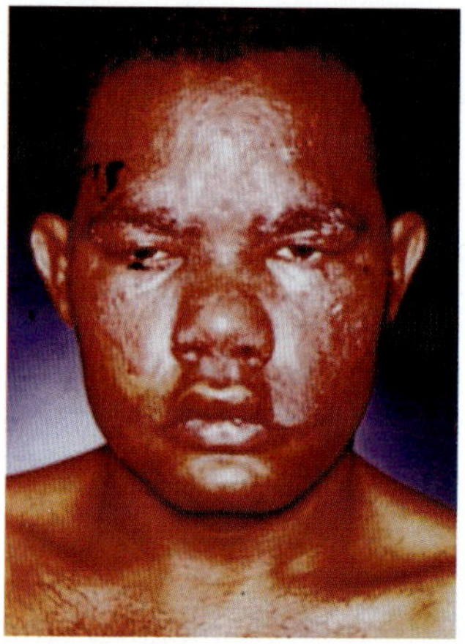

Figure 2-3 Leprosy. The clinical presentation is similar to chronic sarcoid skin lesion of lupus pernio.

M. leprae are either spare or absent. Leprosy may mimic other multisystem disorders with skin and peripheral nervous system involvement.

TL represents T helper cell 1 (Th1) type immune response in which microorganisms is kept to small numbers at the expense of serious tissue damage to the host. While LL represents a Th2 type response where the host tissues are teeming with mycobacteria, and there is little host tissue destruction.[15,16]

FUNGAL GRANULOMAS

Impaired T cell immunity is associated with susceptibility to severe fungal infection.

Bronchocentric Granulomatosis

This is a necrotizing granulomatous inflammatory process that is centered on bronchi and bronchioles and results in focal or complete destruction of their walls. Noninfectious cases predominate, most are a manifestation of allergic bronchopulmonary fungal disease, usually aspergillosis. Bronchocentric granulomatosis is not a specific disease but rather a type of inflammatory reaction pattern due to a variety of noninfectious and infectious causes.

Clinical Presentation

Patients frequently have a history of chronic asthma and may exhibit blood and tissue eosinophilia. The pathogenesis of bronchocentric granulomatosis in asthmatic patients is likely to be related to hypersensitivity against *Aspergillus* antigens. The cause in nonasthmatic patients is unknown.

Bronchocentric granulomatosis is difficult to diagnose for it often causes few respiratory symptoms. The chest radiograph may show infiltrates, nodular lesions, atelectasis, and rarely, adult respiratory distress syndrome (ARDS)-like syndrome.[17]

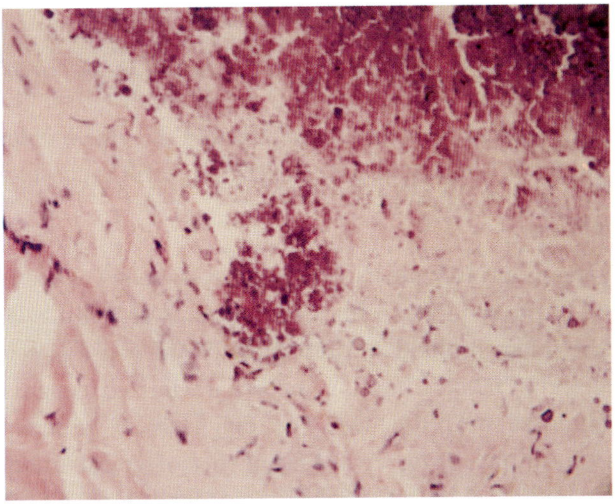

Figure 2-4 Histoplasmosis: granulomas of histoplasmosis are usually round and solitary, sometimes surrounded by sclerosing fibrosis, often containing calcium. *Courtesy* Dr Jelena Stojsic, MD, Service of Pathohistology, Clinical Center Serbia, Department of Pathology, Clinic of Pulmonary Diseases and Clinic of Thoracic Surgery.

Histoplasmosis

Histoplasmosis is a granulomatous infection caused by *Histoplasma capsulatum*, a dimorphic yeast like uninucleate organism, normally found in soil, contaminated by bird's excreta.

Clinical Presentation

Patients with acute pulmonary histoplasmosis often have a history of environmental exposure to sources of infection. Inhalation of spores leads to the lung disease with parenchymal infiltrates and hilar adenopathy. Small outbreaks sometimes occur. The infection may disseminate through the blood or within the lung but spontaneous healing is the most likely outcome. In few cases lately, calcification takes place in the peripheral lesions and they remain permanently visible on the chest X-ray (Figure 2-4).[18]

Accurate diagnosis usually depends on serological tests. Histoplasmin skin test is unlikely to be helpful unless the patients' previous skin test status is known. Moreover, histoplasmin skin testing may itself cause seroconversion. Progressive disseminated histoplasmosis may occur in immunocompromised patients and elderly; immunodiffusion and radioimmunoassay may be needed for accurate diagnosis.[19]

It is difficult to differentiate from TB and sarcoidosis, especially in patients with chronic pulmonary histoplasmosis, which may resemble pulmonary sarcoidosis clinically, pathologically, and radiologically.

PARASITIC GRANULOMATOUS DISEASES

Protozoa (Leishmaniasis)

Leishmania is the cause of a wide spectrum of human diseases. Visceral leishmaniasis (kala azar) is caused by *L. donovani* affecting the entire reticuloendothelial system. Other species of *Leishmania* have mainly dermal or mucosal manifestations.

Clinical Presentation

The infection is common in persons who work at the edge of the forest, which is a natural habitat of the sand flies, although the transmission may also happen by transfusion of the infected blood. Leishmaniasis is the cause of severe interstitial pneumonia. Pulmonary involvement is usually characterized by signs and symptoms of bronchopneumonia or bronchitis. The diagnosis of visceral leishmaniasis depends on an appropriate history, clinical evidence of typical findings of remittent fever, leucopenia, profound anemia, and enlargement of liver and spleen.

The parasites known as Leishman-Donovan bodies are found in the cytoplasm of reticuloendothelial cells or free in the plasma. A serodiagnostic assay for visceral leishmaniasis using a monoclonal antibody has been developed recently.[1] With an increase in human immunodeficiency virus infections in the tropics, kala azar is rising as an important opportunistic infection in patients with acquired immunodeficiency syndrome (Figure 2-5).[20]

Metazoa

Migration of a helminth through the lung may induce a granulomatous reaction of a foreign body type.

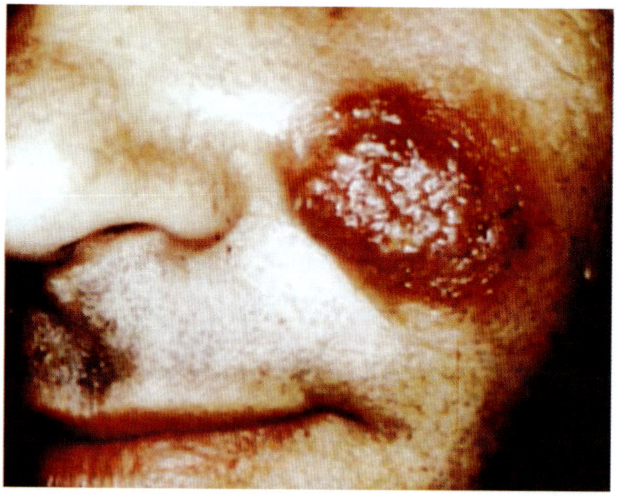

Figure 2-5 Dermal leishmaniasis.

Clinical Presentation

Eosinophilia is characteristic of helmintic infections. Mobilization of eosinophils can be explained by lymphokines released by activated T cells which are chemotactic to eosinophils. The nematodes that cause pulmonary granulomas include *Ascaris lumbricoides, Toxocara canis,* and *Capillaria aerophila.* Patients may present with a visceral larva migrans syndrome, asthmatic syndrome, and eosinophilia. Sometimes, eosinophilia may be absent at the onset of the respiratory symptoms.

Definite diagnosis depends on identifying the larvae in the stools, jejunum, aspirates, sputum, bronchial washings, or transbronchial biopsies. Sometimes, stool samples may be negative for ova or parasites.[1,21]

Trematodes (Schistosomiasis)

The *Schistosoma* or blood flukes are parasitic flat warms. The 3 main species of *Schistosoma* that cause human infection are *S. manosni, S. japonicum,* and *S. haematobium.* They infect more than 200 million people worldwide and the incidence of human infection is further increasing. The disease results from the deposition of eggs by the adult female worms into the host tissue. The eggs induce inflammatory and fibrotic lesions in the host's organs, including the intestines, liver, and lungs.[22]

Clinical Presentation

The clinical manifestations can appear as bronchopulmonary schistosomiasis with bronchitis, bronchiectasis, or asthma due to airway obstruction, widespread arteritis, vessel obstruction, and cor pulmonale. Pulmonary hypertension is reversible. Two types of pathological lesions develop in the lung as a consequences of granuloma formation: extensive parenchymal lesions or periarteritis, fibrosis, and diffuse endarteritis obliterans of pulmonary arterioles.

Severe toxic reactions upon the death of the adult organism in the lungs induce arteriolar thrombosis, necrosis of surrounding lung tissue, and an eosinophilic and giant cell reaction resulting in fibrosis that may calcify.[23]

Occasionally, some eggs may pass from the liver via portal systemic collateral circulation and give rise to granulomas in the lung with pulmonary hypertension and cor pulmonale, and sometimes brain lesion or spinal cord lesion mimicking a space occupying lesion, encephalopathy, or transverse myelitis.[24]

The diagnosis is based on finding the characteristic shistosome eggs in feces, urine, or a biopsy specimen, usually of the rectal mucosa.

BACTERIAL GRANULOMATOUS DISEASES

Brucellosis

Brucella species are zoonotic Gram-negative coccobacilli responsible for bacteriemia in animal hosts but are pathogenic for humans as well. There are 4

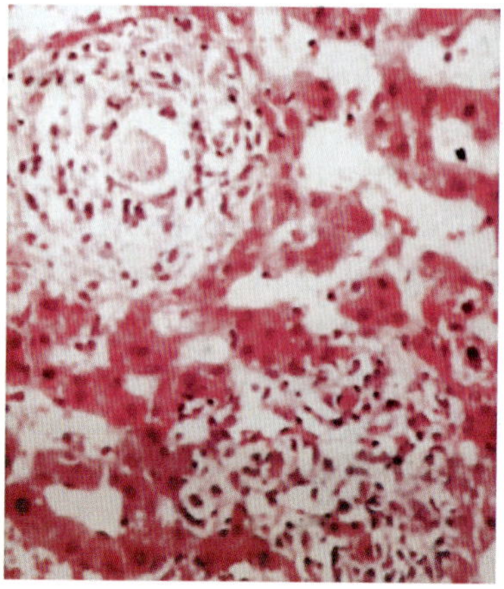

Figure 2-6 *Brucella abortus* infection. The figure shows liver granuloma. These granulomas are poorly formed and lack the elegance of compact, noncaseating sarcoid granulomas.

species of the genus *Brucella* that cause human illness. Each is confined to major animal host: *B. melitensis* to goats, *B. suis* to hogs, *B. abortus* to cattle, and *B. canis* to dogs.

Brucellas are phagocyted by polymorphs, but are capable of remaining viable (particularly *B. melitensis*). Organisms that are not killed localize in mononuclear cells of the reticuloendothelial system. Thus, the prolonged antigenic stimulus leads to lymphokine production and granuloma formation.[1]

Clinical Presentation

Clinical manifestations are described by a range of nonspecific symptoms like chills, relapses of fever, weakness, and vague aches and pains.

The diagnosis is based on specimen isolation from blood, bone marrow, and pus from septic arthritis and osteomyelitis (Figure 2-6).

Tularemia

Tularemia is a zoonotic Gram-negative infection caused by coccobacillus, *Franciella tularensis*. The transmission of an infection occurs by direct contact with animals, contact with water contaminated by their excretions or corpse, investigation of infected tissue, and by insect vectors.

Clinical Presentation

The disease has different manifestations depending on the site of inoculation, but the common features are local ulcer, regional lymphadenopathy, and febrile systemic disease. The host defense mechanisms are not fully understood but the delayed hypersensitivity to tularemia antigen seems to play a role. Septicemic tularemia causes microabscesses in the liver, spleen, and lungs.

The organism is difficult to culture but the diagnosis is based on the organism isolation (culture) of the organism from sputum, gastric lavage fluid, and even blood. There is a danger of laboratory-acquired infection.[1,11,25,26]

GRANULOMATOUS DISEASES OF UNKNOWN CAUSE

Wegener's Granulomatosis

The disease, first described in 1930s, is an organ-specific necrotizing granulomatous vasculitis of the upper and lower respiratory tract together with glomerulonephritis. The histological hallmarks are necrotizing vasculitis of the small arteries and veins together with granuloma formation, intravascular or extravascular. Granuloma formations are rarely seen on renal biopsy.

Clinical Presentation

Besides the classic appearance of the upper and lower respiratory tract involvement and kidney diseases, almost any organ can be involved with vasculitis, granuloma, or both. Wegener's granulomatosis is characterized by a triad consisting of necrotizing granulomatous inflammation of the upper and lower respiratory tract, focal necrotizing vasculitis of small- and medium-caliber vessels, and renal disease in the form of focal necrotizing glomerulitis.[27]

Pulmonary symptoms include cough, hemoptysis, and chest pain. Renal symptoms when present occur after the onset of respiratory symptoms. This disease is presumed to be a manifestation of the delayed hypersensitivity response to an unidentified antigen. Because of the positive response on the therapy with trimethoprine-sulphametoxazole, it is possible that the causative agent may be infectious agent. There are no typical radiological features of Wegner's granulomatosis (Figure 2-7).

A high percentage of patients with Wegener's granulomatosis develop anti-neutrophil cytoplasmic antibody (ANCA). Cytoplasmic-ANCAs (c-ANCAs) are

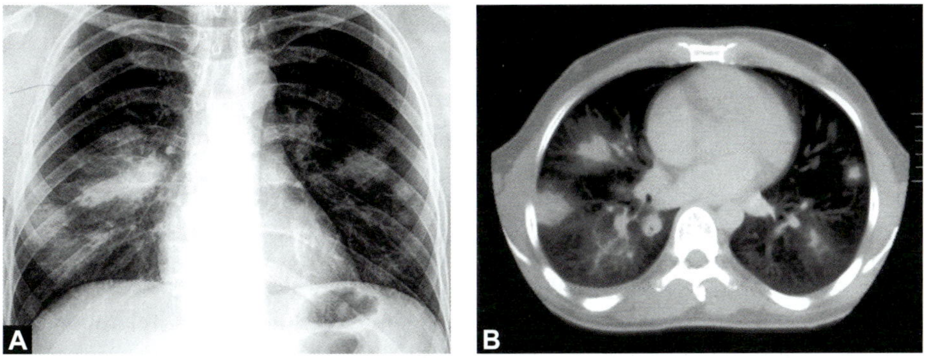

Figure 2-7 Wegener's granulomatosis has no typical radiological presentation. *Courtesy* Professor Dr Dragana Jovanovic and Dr Marta Velinovic, Clinic of Pulmonary Diseases, Clinical Center Belgrade, Serbia, who diagnosed and treated this patient with Wegener granulomatosis.

the predominant ANCAs. The specificity of a positive c-ANCA titer for Wegener's granulomatosis is very high, especially in patients with active glomerulonephritis. However, the diagnosis is based on histological finding of necrotizing granulomatous vasculitis.[28,29]

PULMONARY ALLERGIC GRANULOMATOSIS

Churg-Strauss Syndrome

Churg and Strauss in 1951, described a series of patients with asthma, eosinophilia, and vascular lesions similar to the type seen in polyarteritis nodosa.

Clinical Presentation

The disease may be organized in 3 distinct phases: the prodromal or allergic phase which is characterized by asthma with or without associated allergic rhinitis. Peripheral blood eosinophilia, eosinophilic tissue infiltrates, and/or eosinophil gastroenteritis characterizes the second phase. The third phase is represented with systemic vasculitis.

Histological hallmarks of this disease are necrotizing extravascular granuloma formations and vasculitis of the small arteries and veins.

Bronchoalveolar lavage and pleural fluid demonstrate high eosinophils counts. Most patients have at least one extra pulmonary involvement, i.e., cardiomyopathy, peripheral neuropathy, skin, or central nervous system involvement.[30]

LYMPHOMATOID GRANULOMATOSIS

First described in 1972, this disease is characterized by pulmonary lymphoreticular lesions, angiocentric and angiodestructive.

Clinical Presentation

Pulmonary involvement is the major cause of fatal outcome, but a significant number of patients die from central nervous system involvement.[31]

Pulmonary symptoms include cough, chest pain, and breathlessness. Chest radiograph usually reveals bilateral nodular infiltrates localized in the peripheral parts of the lung parenchyma, so that it may be easily misdiagnosed as metastatic tumors. Other radiological features include cavitation and lesions resembling pneumonia.

SARCOIDOSIS

This granulomatous disease of unknown cause has a worldwide distribution. Almost any organ can be involved, but the majority of patients with sarcoidosis complain of respiratory symptoms. The lungs are involved in more than 90% of patients.

The histological hallmark is noncaseating granuloma composed of epithelioid cells, a few multinucleate giant cells, and a scanty rim of lymphocytes.

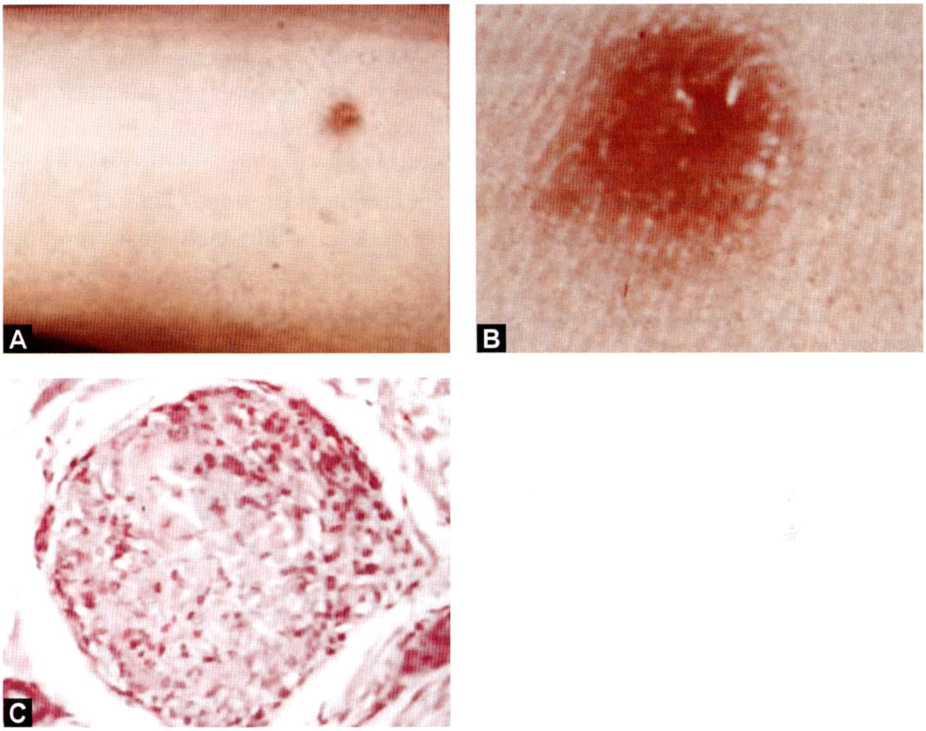

Figure 2-8 Kveim-Siltzbach test. **A,** Nodule appears at the site of inoculation in 4–6 weeks, **B,** magnified view of the nodule, and **C,** the biopsy specimen showing a noncaseating granuloma.

Sarcoidosis is characterized histologically by the presence of non-necrotizing epithelioid granulomas in different organs and systems affecting in the great majority of cases, in the lungs and hilar lymph nodes.[32] Histological hallmark is the "hard" granulomas, in which the epithelioid cell is the dominant element, distributed within the pulmonary interstitium along the pleura and interlobular septa, and around the vasculobronchial axis.[16] Differential diagnosis is made with other granulomatous diseases, such as mycobacterial granulomatosis[33] and berylliosis.[32]

Although non-necrotizing granulomas are the usual finding in sarcoidosis, necrosis does occur. Prior to the widespread use of transbronchial biopsy, necrosis was reported in up to 30% of large biopsy specimens (open lung and lymph node).

Rarely, biopsy material from patients with well-documented sarcoidosis will exhibit extensive necrosis resembling that seen in infectious and other granulomatous processes.

Clinical Presentation

Sarcoidosis most commonly affects young adults. The disease presents commonly with bilateral hilar adenopathy, pulmonary infiltrations, and skin or eye lesions. “It can involve almost any organ system in various combinations, giving rise to many clinical syndromes embracing all branches of medicine."[1]

The diagnosis depends on the clinical and radiological features consistent with the diagnosis of sarcoidosis and the presence of noncaseating granulomas in the tissue biopsy or positive Kveim-Siltzbach test, which is highly specific, and the most useful in differentiating sarcoidosis from all other granulomatous disorders (Figure 2-8).[34,35]

The immunological mechanism of the Kveim-Siltzbach test remains unexplained. It is postulated that the slowly developing sarcoid nodule represents a type of delayed hypersensitivity to an unidentified antigen in the human sarcoid tissue. In patients with active sarcoidosis, the intracutaneous injection of a previously validated saline suspension of human sarcoid spleen or lymph nodes gives rise to a nodule at the site of injection in 4–6 weeks. A biopsy sample of the nodule in a positive reaction should demonstrate characteristic noncaseating granulomas. False-positive reaction to Kveim antigen may occur in patients with TB, lymphoma, or regional enteritis.

ENVIRONMENTAL AND OCCUPATIONAL GRANULOMAS

Hypersensitivity Pneumonitis

This is an inflammatory disorder of the lung parenchyma involving alveolar walls and terminal airways due to repeated inhalation of a variety of organic agents by susceptible host.

This group of lung diseases includes several entities, such as farmers' lung, mushroom workers' lung, bird fanciers' lung, and many others.

The inhalation of organic dust leads to chronic alveolar and interstitial inflammation, granuloma formation, and fibrosis.

Clinical Presentation

The clinical manifestations of the disease vary from patient to patient relating to the frequency and intensity of exposure to the causative agent and perhaps other host factors.

In acute form, it is characterized by cough, fever, chills, malaise, and dyspnea that may occur 6–8 hours after exposure to antigen and usually clear within a few days, if there is no further exposure. The subacute form often appears insidiously over a period of weeks marked by cough, dyspnea, and may progress to cyanosis.

In most patients with acute and subacute form of the disease, symptoms of the disease disappear within days, weeks, or months if the causative agent is no longer inhaled. Transformation to a chronic form of the disease may occur in patients with long antigen exposure. The chronic form may be clinically indistinguishable from pulmonary fibrosis due to different causes.

Diagnostic Approach

An important part of the diagnostic procedure should be performed on any patient with interstitial lung disease, especially if a suggestive exposure of a persistent dry cough, dyspnea with or without wheezing, and malaise. Chest roentgenogram is not specific. It can be normal, even in symptomatic patients. The acute and subacute phase may be associated with nodular infiltrates or diffuse reticulonodular infiltrate.

Lung function tests commonly show restrictive ventilatory impairment, but both the mixed restrictive-obstructive pattern may be present. Diffusing capacity is commonly impaired. Hypoxemia may occur and it is a common feature of the chronic disease.

Diagnosis is confirmed with positive exposure history and/or positive precipitin test against suspected antigens.[11]

BERYLLIOSIS

The natural sources for beryllium are mines in India, the former Soviet Union, some parts of Eastern Europe, and the US. Because of the wide use of beryllium in electronics and airspace industry, the incidence of chronic skin and lung berylliosis due to lower levels of exposure within a prolonged period has sharply increased. The acute form is caused by short-term exposure to high concentrations of beryllium dust, salt, or fumes. Chronic berylliosis is presented as a chronic inflammatory reaction mediated by CD+4 lymphocytes.

Clinical Presentation

The onset of symptoms may appear long after the initial exposure. The symptoms include progressive shortness of breath, chronic cough, weight loss, fatigue, and other symptoms. Chest radiograph may show spotty appearance in both lungs with hilar adenopathy.

Diagnostic Approach

The histological picture may be hard to distinguish from sarcoidosis. Diagnosis depends on the history of exposure, the presence of beryllium in tissues and body fluids, and characteristic histology findings.[36,37]

MISCELLANEOUS PULMONARY GRANULOMATOSIS

Necrotizing Sarcoid Granulomatosis

Necrotizing sarcoid granulomatosis (NSG) is an uncommon condition that primarily involves the lungs, a small number of cases exhibiting extrapulmonary involvement have been reported. The overall prognosis for patients with NSG is excellent.

NSG usually presents radiographically as multiple bilateral nodules in the lung, but may present as a solitary nodule. Evidence of cavitation and hilar lymphadenopathy are occasionally seen. Most patients experience pulmonary symptoms. "Nodular sarcoidosis" is primarily a radiologic diagnosis, the pathologic features of which are not well-documented.[38]

Whipple's Disease

This granulomatous disease is presented with polyarthritis, diarrhea, weight loss, and fever. The affected organs are infiltrated with numerous macrophages containing periodic acid-Schiff positive, diastase resistant glycoprotein. The electronic microscopy reveals the bacteria, *Tropheryma whipplei*. The illness is presented with shrinking lung syndrome, and as granuloma formation often occurs, it might be difficult to differentiate this disease from sarcoidosis.[1,39,40]

Behçet's Disease

Intrathoracic disease is manifested with pulmonary infarctions, pleurisy, pericarditis, and superior vena cava syndrome. Besides pulmonary involvement, orogenital ulceration, uveitis, erythema nodosum, and thrombophlebitis is found. The patient's skin shows characteristic dermatographia which is one of the prominent symptoms of the disease.[1]

Crohn's Regional Enteritis

Intestinal involvement in sarcoidosis is extremely rare and reports are probably examples of Crohn's granulomatous enteritis. Like sarcoidosis, Crohn's disease may be associated with erythema nodosum and iritis. The histology is similar, and except for the clinical symptoms, these 2 granulomatous disorders are difficult to differentiate.[1]

Local Sarcoid-like Granulomatous Reactions

Granulomas may be encountered in association with a variety of malignant neoplasms in the following conditions (Figure 2-9):

- Commonly in Hodgkin disease and non-Hodgkin T cell lymphomas, seminoma of the testis, and ovarian tumors. Some patients with seminoma may develop granulomatous lymphadenitis in nonmetastatic lymph nodes in sites distant from the primary tumor. In Hodgkin disease, granulomas may be seen in liver and spleen which exhibit no evidence of Hodgkin disease involvement
- Uncommonly in carcinomas arising from varied sites and in lymph nodes draining the site of carcinoma
- Coincidental occurrence of a systemic granulomatous disease and a malignant neoplasm.

Drug-induced Pulmonary Granulomas

Drugs that are usually associated with the production of pulmonary granuloma are mineral oil, disodium-cromoglycate, magnesium-trisilicate (known as talc), methotrexate (MTX), and BCG.[1]

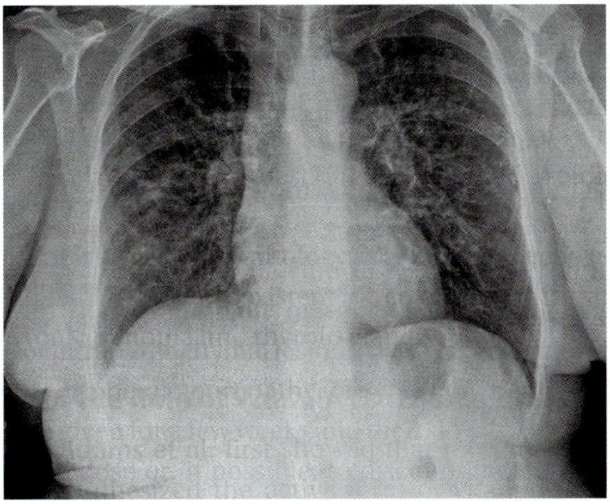

Figure 2-9 Sarcoid-like reaction. The enlargement of the left hilar lymph node—the same side where the breast cancer was treated.

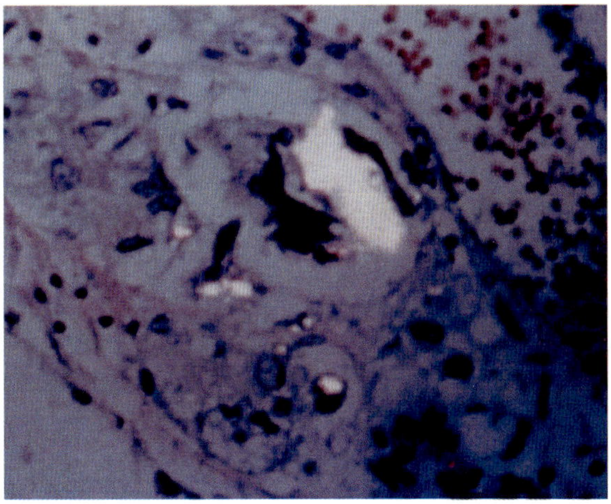

Figure 2-10 Talc-induced granuloma in an intravenous drug addict.

Granulomatous reaction, commonly localized or even fibrosis in the lungs may occur after the inhalation of the oils. Magnesium-trisilicate (talc) which is used in the manufacture of methadone, methylphenidate, and amphetamine pills may initiate granulomatous reaction in pulmonary interstitium (Figure 2-10). BCG recently used as a stimulant of the body immune system to treat various metastatic malignant diseases has also been reported to cause pulmonary granulomas.

MTX has been used in the therapy of the variety of malignant tumors and non-neoplastic diseases, some of them granulomatous (i.e., sarcoidosis). Pneumonitis associated with this drug is well described although the exact mechanism is not known. It is suggested that the pneumonitis related to MTX therapy is related to an immunologically mediated injury rather than a direct toxic effect of MTX.[40]

REFERENCES

1. Sharma OP, Vucinic V. Granulomatous lung diseases in the tropics. *Clin Chest Med.* 2002;23:329-39.
2. Cushley MJ, Davison AG, du Bois RM, Egan J, Flower CD, Gibson GJ, et al. The diagnosis, assessment and treatment of diffuse parenchymal lung disease in adults: British Thoracic Society recommendations. *Thorax.* 1999;54:S1-S30.
3. American Thoracic Society; European Respiratory Society. American Thoracic Society/ European Respiratory Society International Multidisciplinary Consensus Classification of the Idiopathic Interstitial Pneumonias. This joint statement of the American Thoracic Society (ATS), and the European Respiratory Society (ERS) was adopted by the ATS board of directors, June 2001 and by the ERS Executive Committee, June 2001. *Am J Respir Crit Care Med.* 2002;165:277-304.
4. Katzenstein AL. Granulomatous diseases of the lung. In: Katzenstein ALA, editor. Katzenstein and Askins surgical pathology of non-neoplastic lung disease. Philadelphia, USA: WB Saunders; 1997. p. 48-80.
5. Gutierrez EB, Zanett DM, Saldiva PH, Capelozzi VL. Autopsy-proven determinants of death in HIV-infected patients treated for pulmonary tuberculosis in Sao Paulo, Brazil. *Pathol Res Pract.* 2002;198:339-46.
6. Hruban RH, Hutchins GM. Mycobacterial infections. In: Dail DH, Hammar SP, editors. Pulmonary pathology. 2nd ed. New York: Springer-Verlag; 1994. p. 331-50.
7. Lack EE, Connor DH, Chandler FW, Manz HJ. Pathology of infectious diseases. Stamford: Appleton & Lange; 1997. p. 857-68.
8. Muller NL, Fraser RS, Lee KS, Johkoh T. Pulmonary infection. In: Diseases of the lung. Radiologic and pathologic correlations. Philadelphia, USA: Lippincott Williams & Wilkins; 2003. p. 17.
9. Maartens G, Beyers N. Tuberculosis in the Tropics. *Clin Chest Med.* 2002;23:341-50.
10. Waddell R, von Reyn C, Baboo K, Mwing A, Chintu C, Zumla A. The effect of BCG immunization and human immunodeficiency virus infection on skin test ractions to purified protein derivate and Mycobacterium avium sensitin among adults in Zambia. *Int J Tuberc Lung Dis.* 1999:3;255-60.
11. Sharma OP. Diagnosing pulmonary infiltration with eosinophylia syndrome, Part 1. *J Respir Dis.* 2002;23:411-20.
12. Sonnenberg P, Murray J, Glynn JR, Thomas RG, Godfrey-Faussett P, Shearer S. Risk factors for pulmonary disease due to culture positive M tuberculosis or non tuberculosis mycobacteria in South African coal miners. *Eur Resp J.* 2000;15:291-6.
13. Opportunistic mycobacterial pulmonary infection and occupational dust exposure: an investigation in England and Wales. *Tubercle.* 1974;56:295-313.
14. Zumla A, Grange J. Non-tuberculosis mycobacterial infections. *Clin Chest Med.* 2002;23: 369-76.
15. Blake LA, West BC, Lary CH, Todd JR 4th. Environmental nonhuman source of leprosy. *Rev Infect Dis.* 1987;9:562-77.
16. Jindal S, Dattatreya R, Kumar B, Kaur S. Airway hyporesponsive in leprosy—a clinical model of chronic pulmonary denervation, antithetic to asthma (Abstr). *Chest.* 1989;96: 249S.
17. Brooker AS, Sharma OP. Bronchocentric granulomatosis and adult respiratory distress syndrome. *Br J Dis Chest.* 1982;76:189-93.
18. Goodwin RA Jr, Des Prez RM. State of art: histoplasmosis. *Am Rev Respir Dis.* 1978;117: 929-56.

19. Houston S. Tropical respiratory medicine. 3. Histoplasmosis and pulmonary involvement in the tropics. *Thorax.* 1994;49:598-601.
20. Slotar D, Escalante P, Jones BE. Pulmonary manifestation of HIV/AIDS in the tropics. *Clin Chest Med.* 2002;23:355-67.
21. Cook G. Helminth-induced granulomatous disease. In :James DG, Zumla A, editors. The Granulomatous Disorders. Cambridge, UK: Cambridge University Press; 1999. p. 205-11.
22. Cetron MS, Chitsulo L, Sullivan JJ, Pilcher J, Wilson M, Noh J, et al. Schistosomiasis in Lake Malawi. *Lancet.* 1996;348:1274-8.
23. Lanham JG, Churg J. Churg-Straus syndrome. In: Churg A, Churg J, editors. Systemic vasculitides. New York: Igaku-Shoin. 1991. p. 101-20.
24. Sherlock S, Dooley J. Diseases of the liver and biliary system. Oxford, UK: Blackwell Publishing; 2001:481–492.
25. Feldman KA, Enscore RE, Lathrop SL, Matyas BT, McGuill M, Schriefer ME, et al. An outbreak of primary pneumonic tularemia on Martha's Vineyard. *New Engl J Med.* 2001; 345:1601-6.
26. Bevanger L, Maeland JA, Naess AI. Agglutination and antibodies to Francisella tularensis outer membrane antigen in early diagnosis of the disease during an outbreak of tularemia. *J Clin Microbiol.* 1988;26:433-7.
27. Travis WD, Hoffman GS, Leavitt RY, Pass HI, Fauci AS. Surgical pathology of the lung in Wegeners granulomatosis. Review of 87 open lung biopsies from 67 patients. *Am J Surg Pathol.* 1991;15:315-33.
28. Travis WD. Pathology of pulmonary granulomatous vasculitis. *Sarcoidosis Vasc Diffuse Lung Dis.* 1996;13:14-27.
29. Kallenberg CG, Tervaert JW. New treatment of ANCA-associated vasculitis. *Sarc Vasc Diff Lung Dis.* 2000;17:125-9.
30. Savani DM, Sharma OP. Eosinophilic lung disease in the tropics. *Clin Chest Med.* 2002;23:377-96.
31. Katzenstein AL, Carrington CB, Liebow AA. Lymphomatoid granulomatosis: a clinicopathologic study of 152 cases. *Cancer.* 1979;43:360-73.
32. Statement on Sarcoidosis. Joint Statement of the American Thoracic Society (ATS), the European Respiratory Society (ERS) and the World Association of Sarcoidosis and Other Granulomatous Disorders (WASOG) adopted by the ATS Board of Directors and by the ERS Executive Committee, February 1999. *Am J Respir Crit Care Med.* 1999;160:736-55.
33. Rosen Y, Vuletin JC, Pertschurk LP, Silverstein E. Sarcoidosis from the pathologist's vantage point. *Pathol Annu.* 1979;14:405-39.
34. Thomas PD, Hunninghake GW. Current concepts of the pathogenesis of sarcoidosis. *Am Rev Respir Dis.* 1987;135:747-60.
35. Rossman MD, Kern JA, Elias JA, Cullen MR, Epstein PE, Preuss OP, et al. Proliferative response of bronchoalveolar lymphocytes to beryllium. A test for chronic beryllium disease. *Ann Intern Med.* 1988;108:687-93.
36. Infante PF, Newman LS. Beryllium exposure and chronic beryllium disease. *Lancet.* 2004; 363:415-6.
37. Puéchal X. Whipple's disease. *Joint Bone Spine.* 2002;69:133-40.
38. Felipe da Silva AS, da Rosa DC, Capelozzi VL. Interstitial granulomatous pulmonary diseases: a diagnostic approach for the general pathologist. *J Pneumologia.* 2003;29.
39. Sharma OP. Beethoven's illness: Whipple's disease rather thansarcoidosis? *J R Soc Med.* 1994;87:283-5.
40. Limper AH, Rosenow EC 3rd. Drug induced interstitial lung disease. *Curr Opin Pulm Med.* 1996;2:396-404.

CHAPTER

3 Fatigue in Sarcoidosis

INTRODUCTION

Fatigue is a common complaint in general population and also a common symptom in many diseases, such as viral or other infections, hypothyreosis, rheumatoid arthritis, malignant diseases, and anemia.[1-4] Numbers of studies up-to-date have shown fatigue to be one of the most commonly reported complaints of patients suffering from sarcoidosis.[5-8]

The general intent of this chapter is not to solve the problems of fatigue in sarcoidosis, neither to define it as it should be, not even to suggest how to measure it, but to review the possible causes of fatigue observed in the current literature and to illuminate the important problems that the feeling of fatigue is bringing into patients' lives.

HISTORICAL ACCOUNT

Searching the PubMed for "fatigue in sarcoidosis", as many as 46 articles were found. The first published article on the topic fatigue in sarcoidosis was published 40 years ago (1972) in the *Chest* Journal by Sharma[9] and the latest one in July 2011 by Efferich et al.[10] The number of papers, however, increased remarkably during the last decade of this century suggesting that the clinicians treating sarcoidosis patients are aware of the serious problems fatigue can cause.

CLINICAL IMPLICATIONS

Regardless of the published papers, there is still no available definition of fatigue, the most common clinical complaint, in the terms of the clinical practice. There are many synonyms for the word "fatigue" like exhaustion, tiredness, low energy, and weakness. However, all the synonyms describe the sensation of fatigue of a healthy person. The word fatigue indeed originates from the experience of a healthy individual; however, these persons find the same sensation qualitatively completely different once they become sick (Table 3-1).[11]

For clinicians, the duration of fatigue can be divided into: less than 3 months, 3–6 months, and longer than 6 months. In patients with the duration of fatigue longer than 3 months, abdominal, cardiac, musculoskeletal, hematological, and

Table 3-1 Clinical Types of Fatigue in Sarcoidosis[12,13]

Possible clinical manifestations of fatigue in sarcoidosis	
Early morning fatigue	Patients awakes with a feeling of unrest because of joint stuffiness' or muscle pain. This type of fatigue is also seen in patients with auto-immune diseases
Intermittent fatigue	Patients wake-up normally but after a few hours of activity feel tired and exhausted. Throughout the day they need periods of rest
Afternoon fatigue	Patient arises in the morning with adequate energy but feels tired in the early afternoon. These patients evaluate their fatigue as "a flu-like syndrome". They go to bed early and stay in bed until next morning
Post-sarcoidosis chronic fatigue syndrome	Presence of fatigue in persons with the history of sarcoidosis (with the normal chest radiograph and the markers of the disease activity). Main symptoms are widespread myalgia, unbearable fatigue, and depression. Physical signs during the examination are absent. The lack of any objective evidence confuses both the patients and the physicians

neurological system investigations should be performed. In patients with fatigue lasting for more than 6 months, anxiety, family dysfunction, stress, and depression should be considered.[12,13]

POSSIBLE CAUSES OF FATIGUE IN SARCOIDOSIS

General Inflammation and Metabolic (Endocrine) Derangements

Increased inflammation (both systemic and the airways inflammation) has been reported in sarcoidosis.[4] Although increased inflammatory status has also been reported in many chronic illness,[14-16] the relation of proinflammatory mediators (i.e., interleukin-2) and involuntary weight loss and thus the correlation with the sensation of fatigue in sarcoidosis patients has never been analyzed.[17] However, a few case reports with severe weight loss have been reported in sarcoidosis.[18]

On the contrary, patients with high body mass index (overweight) have been described in sarcoidosis with lower fat-free mass over body weight ratio.[19,20]

Male patients with sarcoidosis have been described to have reduced circulating testosterone serum levels related with the sensation of fatigue in many chronic illnesses.[21-23] It has also been described that oxidative stress factors are in correlation with the sensation of fatigue and that antioxidative therapy might be useful in the treatment of fatigue in sarcoidosis.[24,25]

Myopathy

Respiratory Muscle Weakness in Relation to Fatigue in Sarcoidosis

Respiratory muscle weakness has been described in patients with sarcoidosis compared with healthy controls.[4,20,26,27] Reduced inspiratory muscle pressure may be due to granulomatous involvement of the main inspiratory muscle-diaphragm.[28]

The biopsy might be of an important diagnostic value to elucidate the mechanism of respiratory muscle involvement in sarcoidosis, however, not a study on this topic has been performed or published. Although magnetic stimulation of the phrenic nerve might also be helpful in possible explanation of the diaphragmal involvement, it has never been performed in sarcoidosis patients.[29]

The granulomatous involvement of the respiratory muscles should be considered in sarcoidosis patients with complaint of fatigue and dyspnea when the severity of dyspnea does not correlate with the degree of lung function impairments.

Baydur et al. found that forced vital capacity and transfer factor for carbon monoxide were significantly lower in sarcoidosis patients compared to healthy controls, but they did not correlate with the degree of perceived dyspnea. However, low respiratory muscles strength was in correlation with worse dyspnea score on the modified Medical Research Council scale, frequently used as a measure of dyspnea.[26]

It is quite possible that the reduction in respiratory muscles strength, significantly contributed to the feelings of dyspnea and fatigue during usual daily activities in a group of sarcoidosis patients, investigated using daily activity list in a study by Gvozdenovic.[30]

Skeletal Muscle Weakness

Skeletal muscle weakness is assumed to be a part of the granulomatous process in patients with sarcoidosis. Spruit et al.[4] found a significant difference in quadriceps peak torque and handgrip force between patients with sarcoidosis and healthy controls. All patients from this study reported fatigue.

Steroid Induced Myopathy

As already has been described in patients with chronic obstructive pulmonary disease, steroid therapy may also affect respiratory muscles in sarcoidosis patients.[31] Corticosteroid therapy has a significant influence on improvement of granulomatous inflammation in sarcoidosis. However, steroid therapy may also have harmful effects on skeletal muscles force.[32]

In a study of Spruit et al., significant negative correlation was found between quadriceps peak torque and the daily steroid dose in patients who were treated with oral steroid therapy for a period of 6 months prior to the test. Skeletal muscle force, however, did not differ between patients with and without steroid therapy prior to the testing.[4]

Improved skeletal muscle function was reported after the therapy with high doses of oral steroids in patients with sarcoidosis.[33,34]

It seems that the effects of steroid therapy on skeletal muscle function are influenced by the presence of granulomatous inflammation in the muscles.[34]

Sleeping Disorders (Obstructive Sleep Apnea, Restless Legs Syndrome, and Small Fibre Neuropathy)

Sleeping disorders may be a part of the clinical picture of fatigue.[35] Restless leg syndrome (RLS) is probably the most frequent complaint associated with sleep disturbances in sarcoidosis.[36] However, nowadays, it is easily detected by transcranial ultrasound.

The majority of patients with RLS have normal neurological findings on clinical examination and routine neuroimaging.[37,38] Two trascranial ultrasound studies reported a reduction in substantia nigra (SN) echogenicity in 82% of patients with idiopathic RLS and 40% with the secondary RLS. The detectable area of SN was less than 0.1 cm^2. In both groups, the same pathological mechanism was suggested—iron homeostasis disorder in the brain.[39,40]

Pain

Chest pain see the chapter 6 of the possible causes of the chest pain, headache-see chapter 21)

Pain appears to be a substantial problem in sarcoidosis. In a study of Spruit et al.,[4] sarcoidosis patients who complained to be fatigued had positive correlation between quadriceps muscle weakness and Medical Short Form-36 (Section "PAIN"). The lack of energy and feeling of tiredness can possibly explain the variety of pain sensations in sarcoidosis. Therapeutic approach with pain coping regime and rehabilitation program is, therefore, suggested in these patients.[41]

Lack of Exercise

Exercise intolerance has been described in patients with sarcoidosis.[4,42,43] Quadriceps muscle weakness was found to correlate 6-minute walk distance in patients with sarcoidosis who complained of fatigue.[4]

Psychological Factors (Depression)

Although Klonoff and Kleinhenz suggested that sarcoidosis patients as a group does not meet the criteria for clinical depression, awareness of bodily sensations however, was found to be associated with more depressive symptoms and escaping of activities when alone. In relation to psychological factors, fatigue in sarcoidosis may also be related to a perceived stress.[44]

HOW TO MEASURE FATIGUE IN SARCOIDOSIS?

Unfortunately, there is no reliable instrument for measuring fatigue. The sensation of fatigue does not correlate with the objective clinical tests used in everyday practice (chest X-ray, lung function parameters, and routine laboratory tests). Although fatigue has a major influence on the quality of life, from the patients' perspective, doctors seem to be poor adjudicators of this mysterious symptom.

POST-SARCOIDOSIS FATIGUE SYNDROME

To add some more to the confusion called " fatigue in sarcoidosis", doctors treating sarcoidosis patients often notice that the patients frequently complain of fatigue, even when sarcoidosis has come into the clinical remission. Group of Dutch authors[45] in a recent study emphasizes the problem of post-sarcoidosis fatigue as a frequent symptom which can be characterized as a severe long-lasting problem, symptomatically similar to chronic fatigue syndrome (CFS).

Psychological distress and reduced health status are associated with that type of fatigue. Significantly reduced physical activity and muscle weakness were also observed in this group of fatigued patients.

THERAPY

Several case reports of sarcoidosis patients treated with antitumor necrosis factor-α demonstrated a dramatic reduction in fatigue. This kind of drug, however, cannot be given to patients who are suffering exclusively from fatigue without any other evidence of disease activity.[46] Several clinical trials reported positive effects of dexmethylphenidate hydrochloride in treating patients with sarcoidosis associated fatigue. Methylphenidate has already been used in the treatment of fatigue in patients with cancer, HIV infection, and CFS. The drug has also been reported to be effective for medically ill patients with depression, which is an essential part of the clinical picture in patients with fatigue.[47] However, up to date, there are no guidelines for effective treatment of fatigue in sarcoidosis.

CONCLUSION

At the end of this chapter, the "fatigue problems" still remain. It is unclear if muscle weakness is the cause or the consequence of fatigue in some patients. What is the first trigger in the magic circle of granulomatous inflammation and fatigue?

The assessment of fatigue is not an easy task. For clinical studies in sarcoidosis patients, as for the daily practice, the use of health status measures and quality of life measures seems to be essential in order to evaluate patients' subjective well-being.

As a constitutional symptom, fatigue is not reflected in lung function test results or other clinical parameters, but working in daily practice with sarcoidosis patients, it is important to take this symptom seriously. One way of assessing fatigue in the clinical practice may be completion of the fatigue assessment scale (FAS) in regular terms (Table 3-2). Although many of fatigue scales have been used, FAS is the only fatigue questionnaire validated in sarcoidosis patients. This measure might provide physicians with complete information about the nature and extent of the patient's fatigue and the influence of fatigue on their general well-being. This can also bring into focus the sensation of fatigue, and even open the discussion between physicians and patients. Regardless of the insufficient therapy for fatigue, the patients at least can feel that their fatigue problems are taken truthfully.

Table 3-2 The Fatigue Assessment Scale

FAS is a fatigue questionnaire consisting of 10 items: 5 questions reflecting physical fatigue and 5 questions for mental fatigue. The response scale is a 5-point scale (1 never to 5 always). Scores on FAS can range from 10–50, cut-off 22, scores beyond represent fatigue. The following 10 statements refer to how you usually feel. Per statement, you can choose 1 out of 5 answer categories, varying from never to always: 1 = never, 2 = sometimes, 3 = regularly, 4 = often, and 5 = always. Items 4 and 10 require reversed scoring. The scale score is calculated by summing all item scores

Statements	*Never*	*Sometimes*	*Regularly*	*Often*	*Always*
I am bothered by fatigue	1	2	3	4	5
I get tired very quickly	1	2	3	4	5
I don't do much during the day	1	2	3	4	5
I have enough energy for everyday life	1	2	3	4	5
Physically I feel exhausted	1	2	3	4	5
I have problems getting started	1	2	3	4	5
I have problems thinking clearly	1	2	3	4	5
I feel no desire to do anything	1	2	3	4	5
Mentally I feel exhausted	1	2	3	4	5
When I am doing something I can concentrate quite well	1	2	3	4	5

FAS, fatigue assessment scale.
The FAS is also available online in the e-version; fatigue scores (mental, physical, and total fatigue score) can be calculated immediately at www.ildcare.eu/.

REFERENCES

1. Hinz A, Fleischer M, Brähler E, Wirtz H, Bosse-Henck A. Fatigue in patients with sarcoidosis, compared with the general population. *Gen Hosp Psychiatry.* 2011;33:462-8.
2. Lacasse Y, Brosseau L, Milne S, Martin S, Wong E, Guyatt GH, et al. Pulmonary rehabilitation for chronic obstructive pulmonary disease. *Cochrane Database Syst Rev.* 2002:CD003793.
3. De Vries J, Michielsen HJ, Van Heck GL, Drent M. Measuring fatigue in sarcoidosis: the Fatigue Assessment Scale (FAS). Br J Health Psychol. 2004;9:279-91.
4. Spruit MA, Thomeer MJ, Gosselink R, Troosters T, Kasran A, Debrock AJ, et al. Skeletal muscle weakness in patients with sarcoidosis and its relationship with exercise intolerance and reduced health status. *Thorax.* 2005;60:32-8.
5. Michielsen HJ, Drent M, Peros-Golubicic T, De Vries J. Fatigue is associated with quality of life in sarcoidosis patients. *Chest.* 2006;130:989-94.
6. Baughman RP, Sparkman BK, Lower EE. Six-minute walk test and health status assessment in sarcoidosis. *Chest.* 2007;132:207-13.
7. De Vries J, Drent M. Quality of life and health status in sarcoidosis: a review of the literature. *Clin Chest Med.* 2008;29:525-32, ix.
8. De Kleijn WP, De Vries J, Lower EE, Elfferich MD, Baughman RP, Drent M. Fatigue in sarcoidosis: a systematic review. *Curr Opin Pulm Med.* 2009;15:499-506.
9. Sharma OP. Fatigue, chest pain, and left testicular discomfort in a 28-year-old man. *Chest.* 1972;61;77-8.

10. Elfferich MD, De Vries J, Drent M. Type D or 'distressed' personality in sarcoidosis and idiopathic pulmonary fibrosis. *Sarcoidosis Vasc Diffuse Lung Dis.* 2011;28:65-71.
11. Glaus A, Crow R, Hammond S. A qualitative study to explore the concept of fatigue/ tiredness in cancer patients and in healthy individuals. *Eur J Cancer Care.* 1996;5:8-23.
12. Sharma OP. Fatigue and sarcoidosis. *Eur Resp J.* 1999;13:713-4.
13. James DG. Complications of sarcoidosis. *Sarcoidosis.* 1993;10:1-3.
14. Di Francia M, Barbier D, Mege JL, Orehek J. Tumor necrosis factor-alpha levels and weight loss in chronic obstructive pulmonary disease. *Am J Respir Crit Care Med.* 1994; 150:1453-5.
15. Libera LD, Vescovo G. Muscle wastage in chronic heart failure, between apoptosis, catabolism and altered anabolism: a chimaeric view of inflammation? *Curr Opin Clin Nutr Metab Care.* 2004;7:435-441.
16. Nelson KA, Walsh D. The cancer anorexia-cachexia syndrome: a survey of the Prognostic Inflammatory and Nutritional Index (PINI) in advanced disease. *J Pain Symptom Manage.* 2002;24:424-8.
17. Spruit MA, Wouters EFM, Gosselink R. Rehabilitation programmes in sarcoidosis: a multidisciplinary approach. *Eur Respir Mon.* 2005;32:316-26.
18. Friedman M, Ali MA, Borum ML. Gastric sarcoidosis: a case report and review of the literature. *South Med J.* 2007;100:301-3.
19. Drent M, Wirnsberger RM, De Vries J, Dieijen-Visser MP, Wouters EF, Schols AM. Association of fatigue with an acute phase response in sarcoidosis. *Eur Respir J.* 1999; 13:718-22.
20. Wirnsberger RM, Drent M, Hekelaar N, Breteler MH, Drent S, Wouters EF, et al. Relationship between respiratory muscle function and quality of life in sarcoidosis. *Eur Respir J.* 1997;10:1450-5.
21. Adler RA, Funkhouser HL, Petkov VI, Berger MM. Glucocorticoid-induced osteoporosis in patients with sarcoidosis. *Am J Med Sci.* 2003;325:1-6.
22. Casaburi R, Bhasin S, Cosentino L, Porszasz J, Somfay A, Lewis MI, et al. Effects of testosterone and resistance training in men with chronic obstructive pulmonary disease. *Am J Respir Crit Care Med.* 2004;170:870-8.
23. Wagner GJ, Rabkin JG, Rabkin R. Testosterone as a treatment for fatigue in HIV+ men. *Gen Hosp Psychiatry.* 1998;20:209-13.
24. Boots AW, Drent M, Swennen EL, Moonen HJ, Bast A, Haenen GR. Antioxidant status associated with inflammation in sarcoidosis: a potential role for antioxidants. *Respir Med.* 2009;103:364-72.
25. Vucinic V, Kotur-Stevuljic J, Vukovic M, Videnovic-Ivanov J, Filipovic S, Gvozdenovic B, et al. Coexistence between fatigue and oxidative stress – total antioxidative status (TAS) in patients with sarcoidosis. *Sarcoidosis Vasc Diffuse Lung Dis.* 2011;28. Abstract E6.
26. Baydur A, Alsalek M, Louie SG, Sharma OP. Respiratory muscle strength, lung function, and dyspnea in patients with sarcoidosis. *Chest.* 2001;120:102-8.
27. Baydur A, Pandya K, Sharma OP, Kanel GC, Carlson M. Control of ventilation, respiratory muscle strength, and granulomatous involvement of skeletal muscle in patients with sarcoidosis. *Chest.* 1993;103:396-402.
28. Pringle CE, Dewar CL. Respiratory muscle involvement in severe sarcoid myositis. *Muscle Nerve.* 1997;20:379-81.
29. Man WD, Moxham J, Polkey MI. Magnetic stimulation for the measurement of respiratory and skeletal muscle function. *Eur Respir J.* 2004;24:846-60.
30. Gvozdenovic B, Mihailovic-Vucinic V, Ilic-Dudvarski A, Zugic V, Judson M. Differences in symptom severity and health status impairment between patients with pulmonary and pulmonary plus extra pulmonary sarcoidosis. *Respir Med.* 2008;102:1636-42.

31. Decramer M, Lacquet LM, Fagard R, Rogiers P. Corticosteroids contribute to muscle weakness in chronic airflow obstruction. *Am J Respir Crit Care Med.* 1994;150:11-6.
32. Barry SC, Gallagher CG. Corticosteroids and skeletal muscle function in cystic fibrosis. *J Appl Physiol.* 2003;95:1379-84.
33. Hearth-Holmes M, Campbell GD Jr. Muscle weakness, fatigue, and joint pain in a 52-year-old woman. *Chest.* 1995;108:563-4.
34. Mozaffar T, Lopate G, Pestronk A. Clinical correlates of granulomas in muscle. *J Neurol.* 1998;245:519-24.
35. Drent M, Verbraecken J, van der Grinten C. Wouters. Fatigue associated with obstructive sleep apnea in a patient with sarcoidosis. *Respiration.* 2000;67:337-40.
36. Vucinic V, Mijailovic M, Sternic N, Vukovic M, Videnovic J, Filipovic S, et al. Trascranial ultrasound (TCS) in sarcoidosis-relation to fatigue, depression and anxiety. *Sarcoidosis Vasc Diffuse Lung Dis.* 2011;28. Abstract E7.
37. Allen RP, Barket PB, Wehr F, Song HK, Earley CJ. MRI measurement of brain iron in patients with restless legs syndrome. *Neurology.* 2001;56:263-5.
38. Allen RP, Picchietti D, Hening WA, Trenkwalder C, Walters AS, Montplaisi J, et al. Restless legs syndrome: diagnostic criteria, special considerations, and epidemiology. A report from the restless legs syndrome diagnosis and epidemiology workshop at the National Institutes of Health. *Sleep Med.* 2003;4:101-19.
39. Schmidauer C, Sojer M, Seppi K, Stockner H, Högl B, Biedermann B, et al. Transcranial ultrasound shows nigral hypoechogenicity in restless legs syndrome. *Ann Neurol.* 2005; 58:630-4.
40. Godau J, Schweitzer KJ, Liepelt I, Gerloff Ch, Berg D. Substantia nigra hyperechogenicity: definition and findings in restless legs syndrome. *Mov Disord.* 2007;22:187-92.
41. Hoitsma E, de Vries J, Santen-Hoeufft M, Faber CG, Drent M. Impact of pain in a Dutch sarcoidosis patient population. *Sarcoidosis Vasc Diffuse Lung Dis.* 2003;20:33-9.
42. Sietsema KE, Kraft M, Ginzton L, Sharma OP. Abnormal oxygen uptake responses to exercise in patients with mild pulmonary sarcoidosis. *Chest.* 1992;102:838-45.
43. Delobbe A, Perrault H, Maitre J, Robin S, Hossein-Foucher C, Wallaert B, et al. Impaired exercise response in sarcoid patients with normal pulmonary function. *Sarcoidosis Vasc Diffuse Lung Dis.* 2002;19:148-53.
44. Klonoff EA, Kleinhenz ME. Psychological factors in sarcoidosis: the relationship between life stress and pulmonary function. *Sarcoidosis.* 1993;10:118-24.
45. Korenromp HEI, Heijnen JC, Vogels JO, van den Bosch MMJ, Grutters CJ. Characterization of chronic fatigue in sarcoidosisin clinical remission. *Chest.* 2011;140:441-7.
46. De Vries J, Drent M. Quality of life and health status in sarcoidosis. In: Baughman RP, editor. Sarcoidosis, New York: Marcel Dekker; 2005.
47. Lower E, Harman S, Baughman RP. Double-blind, randomized trial of treatment of sarcoidosis-associated fatigue dexmethylphenidate hydrochloride for the treatment of sarcoidosis associated fatigue. *Chest.* 2008;133;1189-95.

CHAPTER

4 Cough in Sarcoidosis

INTRODUCTION

Pulmonary manifestations are generally the predonimal preseutations in more than 90% of sarcoidosis patients. Respiratory symptoms: dyspnea, dry cough, and chest pain occur in one-third to one-half of patients with sarcoidosis.[1]

One of the major symptom of sarcoidosis, cough, is seen in 40–80% of symptomatic patients with sarcoidosis.[2]

The pathogenesis of cough in sarcoidosis is not definitely elucidated, however, certain factors play a significant role into developing persistent cough in sarcoidosis.

POSSIBLE CAUSES OF CHRONIC COUGH IN SARCOIDOSIS

The possible causes of chronic cough in sarcoidosis are:

- Airway involvement
- Parenchymal lesions
- Endobronchial sarcoidosis
- Extrinsic airways compression by the enlarged lymph nodes
- Airway obstruction.

Prior to concluding that sarcoidosis is the essential cause of cough, other common conditions should be excluded as contributing or primary causes of cough (i.e., upper airway cough syndrome and gastroesophageal reflux disease).[3]

Airway Involvement Causing Cough in Sarcoidosis

It is already mentioned that airway involvement might be the cause of dyspnea in sarcoidosis. Here, we will point out the airway involvement as the cause of chronic hacking cough. According to the anatomical localization of sarcoid lesions, the involvement of supraglotic airways (seen in approximately 6% of patients with sarcoidosis) can lead to irritating cough besides other symptoms like dyspnea, stridor, dysphonia, dysphagia, hyponasal speech, or retronasal obstruction. Besides endoscopy, flow-volume curves are helpful in establishing the diagnosis.[4-9]

Involvement of trachea and of the major bronchia lead to chronic cough as the main symptom of this localization of sarcoid lesions. It can rarely cause obstruction

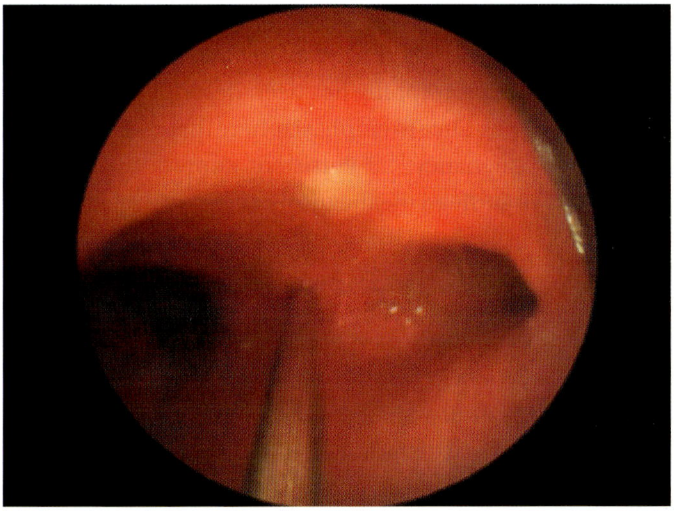

Figure 4-1 Compression by enlarged lymph nodes in sarcoidosis (endoscopic view). Possible cause of predominantly dry, hacking cough. In the same patient, there was evidence of granulomatous lesion on mucosa (white node) of the central airway right above the central carina which was enlarged by extramural compression of the lymph nodes. *Courtesy:* Professor Dragan Mandaric, Dr Emilija Sudjic-Bukurov. Department of Bronchology, Clinic of Pulmonary Diseases, Clinical Center Belgrade, Serbia.

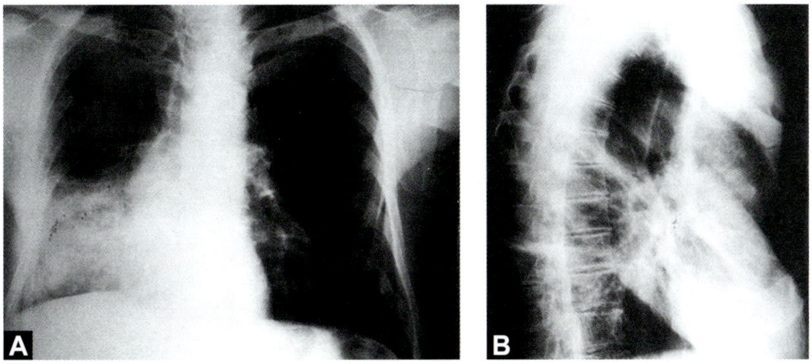

Figure 4-2 Right middle lobe syndrome in sarcoidosis (composite). As in other conditions, when occurs right, middle lobe syndrome in sarcoidosis may be the cause of chronic long lasting cough.

of the involved airways.[10] Besides bronchoscopy, which is all unavoidable procedure in establishing correct diagnosis, flow-volume curves are helpful in assessing the severity of central airway stenosis.[11]

Extrinsic compression of the central airways by enlarged mediastinal lymph nodes is rare but cause of dry cough in sarcoidosis is possible (Figure 4-1). In these patients, bronchoscopy and/or endobronchial ultrasound-guided transbronchial fine-needle aspiration leads to diagnosis. Differential diagnosis to lymphoma is important.[10] Right middle lobe syndrome is also described in sarcoidosis (Figure 4-2). As in other conditions, when occurs, right middle lobe syndrome in sarcoidosis may be the cause of chronic long-lasting cough.[12] Small airway involvement (small airway disease) frequently correlating with air trapping has been described in sarcoidosis.[13]

It is of great clinical importance to emphasize here that endobronchial sarcoidosis can mimic asthma or malignancy.[14-16] Persistent nonproductive cough is a major symptom that can lead or mislead the diagnosis.

Airway Obstruction in Sarcoidosis

Although restrictive pattern of pulmonary function tests has been described in sarcoidosis with reducing volumes, i.e., vital capacity (VC) and total lung capacity,[17-19] airway obstruction with reduced forced expiratory volume in 1 second (FEV1) and expiratory flow rates occurs in 28–50% of patients with pulmonary sarcoidosis. Airway obstruction occurs at all stages with its frequency increasing from stage 1 to stage 4.[20]

Airway obstruction in sarcoidosis is reported to be associated with increased morbidity, underlined respiratory symptoms (i.e., chronic cough), and even increased mortality risk (Figure 4-3). Viskum and Vestibo pointed out that sarcoidosis patients with an FEV1/FEV ratio <70% predicted value had increased mortality risk of 1,9 compared with patients with FEV1/VC ≥70% of predicted value.[21]

Airway obstruction can be either completely or partially reversed by steroid therapy and the improvement is always accompanied with the attenuation or complete disappearance of respiratory symptoms. Although oral corticosteroid therapy may lead to symptomatic improvement, it is also associated with

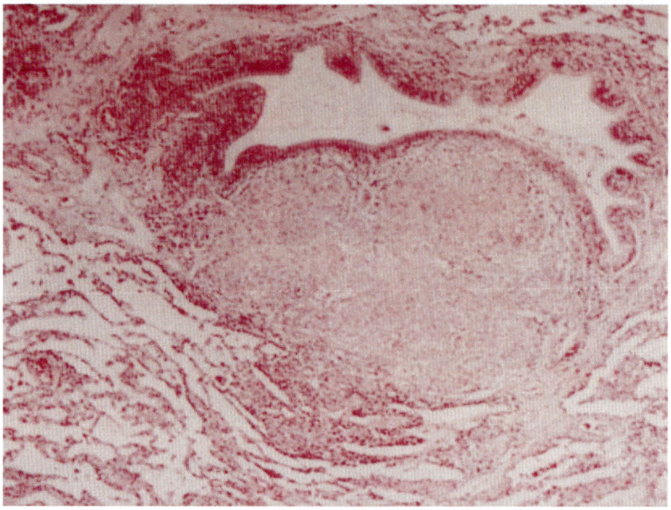

Figure 4-3 An open lung biopsy specimen showing a sarcoid granuloma in the bronchial wall causing obstruction. The patient had lung function changes consistent with airway obstruction. Airway obstruction in sarcoidosis is common and may remain asymptomatic or produce severe cough.

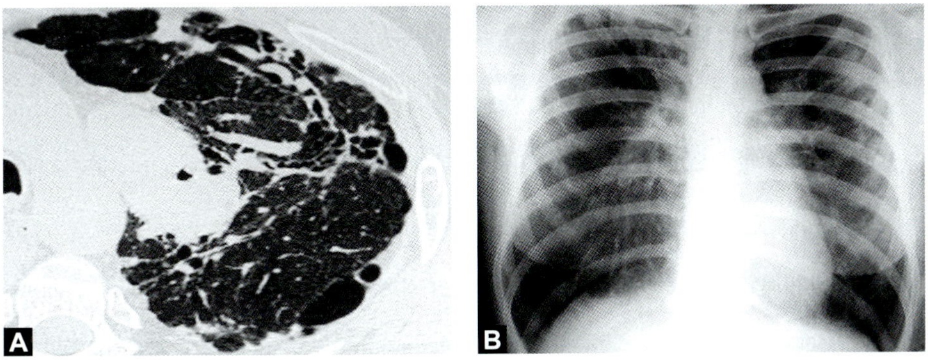

Figure 4-4 **A,** Distortion of the airways caused by pulmonary fibrosis [computed tomography (CT) scan—right] (composite). The figure represents CT scan in patient with chronic multisystem sarcoidosis. The diagnosis of sarcoidosis was established 10 years ago. **B,** Chest X-ray —left. The patient also had skin sarcoidosis and sarcoidosis of the bone. Last year she died at the age of 61 years due to respiratory insufficiency.

significant side effects and individualized analyzes of the overall benefit and risk is necessary.[3,22]

Airway obstruction in sarcoidosis has different mechanisms. Bronchoscopy and thoracic computed tomography (CT) scan are necessary diagnostic procedures to assess which of the possible mechanism is involved (Figure 4-4).[23]

CT scan represents linear opacities associated with bronchial distortion. Bullae are also clearly visible in the periphery of the lung parenchyma.

POSSIBLE CAUSES OF AIRWAY OBSTRUCTION IN SARCOIDOSIS AND DIAGNOSTIC PROCEDURES

Narrowing of the bronchial walls is either caused by intramural granulomatous lesions or fibrotic scarring. Diagnosis is established on bronchoscopy or CT scans:[24]

- Distortion of the airways caused by pulmonary fibrosis (diagnosis is suggested by CT scans)[24]
- Compression by enlarged lymph nodes (diagnostic procedures chest X-ray and CT scans)[25]
- Small airway disease is also suggested by CT scans: (bronchial thickening, small airway narrowing, and patchy air trapping)[11,22,26-29]
- Bronchial hyperreactivity—increased airway sensitivity to metacholine is common in patients with sarcoidosis, and is often clinically manifested as chronic, persistent, hacking cough, and wheezing; the hyperreactivity is probably due to granulomatous inflammation of the bronchial mucosa.[18,29-32]

REFERENCE

1. Statement on sarcoidosis. Joint Statement of the American Thoracic Society (ATS), the European Respiratory Society (ERS) and the World Association of Sarcoidosis and Other

Granulomatous Disorders (WASOG) adopted by the ATS Board of Directors and by the ERS Executive Committee, February 1999. *Am J Respir Crit Care Med.* 1999;160:736-55.

2. Sharma SK, Mohan A, Guleria JS. Clinical characteristics, pulmonary function abnormalities and outcome of prednisolone treatment in 106 patients with sarcoidosis. *J Assoc Physicians India.* 2001;49:697-704.
3. Brown KK. Chronic cough due to chronic interstitial pulmonary diseases: ACCP evidence-based clinical practice guidelines. *Chest.* 2006;129:180S–185S.
4. Hunninghake GW, Costabel U, Ando M, Baughman R, Cordier JF, du Bois R, et al. ATS/ERS/WASOG statement on sarcoidosis: American Thoracic Society/European Respiratory Society/World Association of Sarcoidosis and other Granulomatous Disorders. *Sarcoidosis Vasc Diffuse Lung Dis.* 1999;16:149-73.
5. Rottoli P, Bargagli E, Chidichimo C, Nuti D, Cintorino M, Ginanneschi C, et al. Sarcoidosis with upper respiratory tract involvement. *Respir Med.* 2006;100:253-7.
6. Sharma OP. Sarcoidosis of the upper respiratory tract: selected cases emphasizing diagnostic and therapeutic difficulties. *Sarcoidosis Vasc Diffuse Lung Dis.* 2002;19:227-33.
7. Braun JJ, Gentine A, Pauli G. Sinonasal sarcoidosis: review and report of fifteen cases. *Laryngoscope.* 2004;114:1960-3.
8. Rizzato G, Palmieri G, Agrati AM, Zanussi C. The organ-specific extrapulmonary presentation of sarcoidosis: a frequent occurrence but a challenge to an early diagnosis; a 3-year-long prospective observational study. *Sarcoidosis Vasc Diffuse Lung Dis.* 2004; 21:119-26.
9. Baughman RP, Teirstein AS, Judson MA, Rossman MD, Yeager H Jr, Bresnitz EA, et al; Case Control Etiologic Study of Sarcoidosis (ACCESS) research group. Clinical characteristics of patients in a case control study of sarcoidosis. *Am J Respir Crit Care Med.* 2001;164:1885-9.
10. Polychronopoulos VS, Prakash UB. Airway involvement in sarcoidosis. *Chest.* 2009;136; 1371-80.
11. Harrison BD, Shaylor JM, Stokes TC, Wilkes AR. Airflow limitation in sarcoidosis -- a study of pulmonary function in 107 patients with newly diagnosed disease. *Respir Med.* 1991;85:59-64.
12. Mendelson DS, Norton K, Cohen BA, Brown LK, Rabinowitz JG. Bronchial compression: an unusual manifestation of sarcoidosis. *J Comput Assist Tomogr.* 1983;7:892-4.
13. Miller A, Teirstein AS, Jackler I, Chuang M, Siltzbach LE. Airway function in chronic pulmonary sarcoidosis with fibrosis. *Am Rev Respir Dis.* 1974;109:179-89.
14. Mixides G, Guy E. Can Sarcoidosis confined to the airway masquerading as asthma. *Respir J.* 2003;10:114-6.
15. Corsello BF, Lohaus GH, Funahashi A. Endobronchial mass lesion due to sarcoidosis: complete resolution with corticosteroids. *Thorax.* 1983;38:157-8.
16. Abramowicz MJ, Ninane V, Depierreux M, de Francquen P, Yernault JC. Tumour-like presentation of pulmonary sarcoidosis. *Eur Respir J.* 1992;5:1286-7.
17. Sharma OP, Johnson R. Airway obstruction in sarcoidosis: a study of 122 nonsmoking black American patients with sarcoidosis. *Chest.* 1988;94:333-6.
18. Subramanian I, Flaherty K, Martinez F. Pulmonary function testing in sarcoidosis. In: Baughman RP, editor. Sarcoidosis. New York: Taylor and Francis Group; 2006. p. 415-32.
19. McCann BG, Harrison BD. Bronchiolar narrowing and occlusion in sarcoidosis: correlation of pathology with physiology. *Respir Med.* 1991;85:65-7.
20. Lamberto C, Saumon G, Loiseau P, Battesti JP, Georges R. Respiratory function in recent pulmonary sarcoidosis with special reference to small airways. *Bull Eur Physiopathol Respir.* 1985;21:309-15.

21. Viskum K, Vestbo J. Vital prognosis in intrathoracic sarcoidosis with special reference to pulmonary function and radiological stage. *Eur Respir J.* 1993;6:339–53.
22. Lavergne F, Clerici C, Sadoun D, Brauner M, Battesti JP, Valeyre D. Airway obstruction in bronchial sarcoidosis: outcome with treatment. *Chest.* 1999;116:1194-9.
23. Chambellan A, Turbie P, Nunes H, Brauner M, Battesti JP, Valeyre D. Endoluminal stenosis of proximal bronchi in sarcoidosis: bronchoscopy, function, and evolution. *Chest.* 2005;127:472-81.
24. Miller A, Brown LK, Sloane MF, Bhuptani A, Teirstein AS. Cardiorespiratory responses to incremental exercise in sarcoidosis patients with normal spirometry. *Chest.* 1995;107:322-9.
25. Lynch JP III, Kazerooni EA, Gay SE. Pulmonary sarcoidosis. *Clin Chest Med.* 1997;18:755-85.
26. Gleeson FV, Traill ZC, Hansell DM. Evidence of expiratory CT scans of small-airway obstruction in sarcoidosis. *AJR Am J Roentgenol.* 1996;166:1052-4.
27. Radwan L, Grebska E, Koziorowski A. Small airways function in pulmonary sarcoidosis. *Scand J Respir Dis.* 1978;59:37-43.
28. Levinson RS, Metzger LF, Stanley NN, Kelsen SG, Altose MD, Cherniack NS, et al. Airway function in sarcoidosis. *Am J Med.* 1977;62:51-9.
29. Mihailovic-Vucinic V, Zugic V, Videnovic-Ivanov J. New observations on pulmonary function changes in sarcoidosis. *Curr Opin Pulm Med.* 2003;9:436-41.
30. Benatar SR, Clark TJ. Pulmonary function in a case of endobronchial sarcoidosis. *Am Rev Respir Dis.* 1974;110:490-6.
31. Ohrn MB, Skold CM, van Hage-Hamsten M, Sigurdardottir O, Zetterstrom O, Eklund A. Sarcoidosis patients have bronchial hyperreactivity and signs of mast cell activation in their bronchoalveolar lavage. *Respiration.* 1995;62:136-42.
32. Bechtel JJ, Starr T III, Dantzker DR, Bower JS. Airway hyperreactivity in patients with sarcoidosis. *Am Rev Respir Dis.* 1981;124:759-61.

CHAPTER

5 Dyspnea in Sarcoidosis

INTRODUCTION

Defined as difficult or labored breathing, or shortness of breath, dyspnea is a common symptom and sign of serious disease of the airway, lungs, or heart. However, dyspnea may be also caused by nonorganic reasons like anxiety and depression.

HISTORIC ACCOUNT

The word dyspnea originates from the Greek language meaning difficult breathing ("dys"—difficulty and "pnoia"—breathing). The ancient Greek philosopher once wrote "A human being is only breath and shadow"—Sophocles.[1]

CLINICAL IMPORTANCE

As a common symptom in many cardiac or pulmonary disease, dyspnea can be effectively managed in the office by family physicians using easily performed tests that can provide valuable information considering the diagnosis, i.e., careful detailed history, physical examination, chest radiographs, electrocardiograph, and screening spirometry.

In sarcoidosis, dyspnea is the most common symptom and clinical presentation from an early stage of lung involvement to advanced disease.

The causes of dyspnea in sarcoidosis are variable (Table 5-1):

- Lesions of the airways
- Lesions of the lung parenchyma
- Lesions of the pleura
- Lesions of the respiratory muscles
- Lesions present in sarcoidosis of the upper airways and laryngeal lesions
- Pulmonary vascular involvement—pulmonary arterial hypertension (PAH).

Lesions of the Airways Causing Dyspnea

Airway involvement in sarcoidosis may occur in all stages. The involvement of the airways as detected by patient's history, clinical presentations, pulmonary function testing, imaging techniques, bronchoscopy, and/or airway mucosal biopsy has been observed in approximately two-thirds of sarcoidosis patients. Obstructive

Table 5-1 Possible Causes of Dyspnea in Sarcoidosis[4-18]

Cause	*Suggested diagnostic procedures to verify the cause*
Lesions of the airways structural lesions	
• Mucosal (edema, erythema, and nodular lesions)	Bronchoscopy
• Bronchial obstruction	
• Stenosis	Bronchoscopy + HRCT
• Airway distortion	HRCT
• Compression of the airway (significant adenopathy)	CT/HRCT
• Laryngeal involvement	Laryngoscopy
• SURT nasal or oral passages lesions	Rhinopharyngoscopy
Functional lesions of the airways	
• Bronchial hyperreactivity in sarcoidosis	Pulmonary function tests
• Obstructive sleep apnea	Sleep tests
Lesions of the lung parenchyma	
Pleural lesions	Pleural biopsy, pleuroscopy
Lesions of the respiratory muscles	Pulmonary function tests
Pulmonary vascular involvement—pulmonary arterial hypertension	Right heart catheterization, Doppler echocardiography

CT, computed tomography; HRCT, high resolution computed tomography; SURT, sarcoidosis of the upper respiratory tract.

airway disease has been noted in 63% of African-American patients with sarcoidosis compared to lower percents in white European and American patients and in patients in Japan. The entire airway system may be affected in sarcoidosis (from nasal and oral passages to terminal bronchioles) leading to dyspnea and cough as prominent clinical symptoms.

Clinicians should be aware of the possibility of the airway involvement in sarcoidosis, especially in patients with persistent dyspnea or chronic cough that did not respond to steroid therapy.

Lesions of the Lung Parenchyma Causing Dyspnea

In some patients with sarcoidosis, advanced fibrotic parenchymal disease may lead to obstructive airway distraction, bullous changes, peribronchial, or peribronchiolar fibrosis.[19-21]

From 1988 to 2007, sarcoidosis-related mortality rates increased significantly; the underlying cause of death in most patients with sarcoidosis was pulmonary fibrosis or cardiac involvement.[22] Pulmonary parenchymal infiltrates are present in 20–50% of sarcoidosis patients with or without BHLA. The infiltrates commonly involve the upper and mid lung zones (Figure 5-1).[3,23,24]

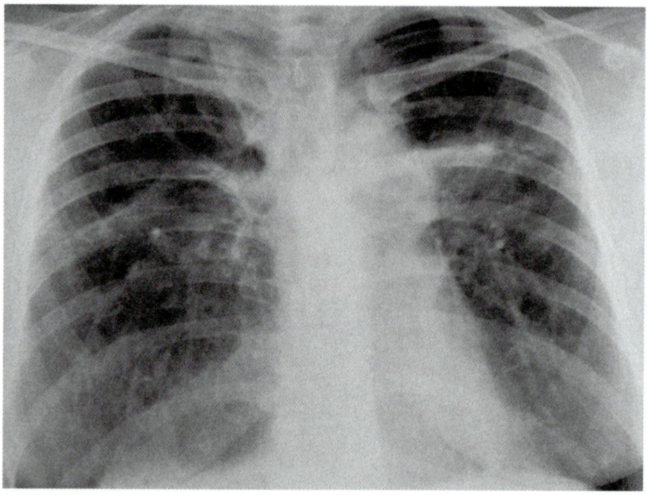

Figure 5-1 Pulmonary parenchymal infiltrates are present in 20–50% of sarcoidosis patients with or without bilateral hilar adenopathy. The infiltrates commonly involve the upper and mid lung zones. The presence of parenchymal lesions may cause dyspnea.

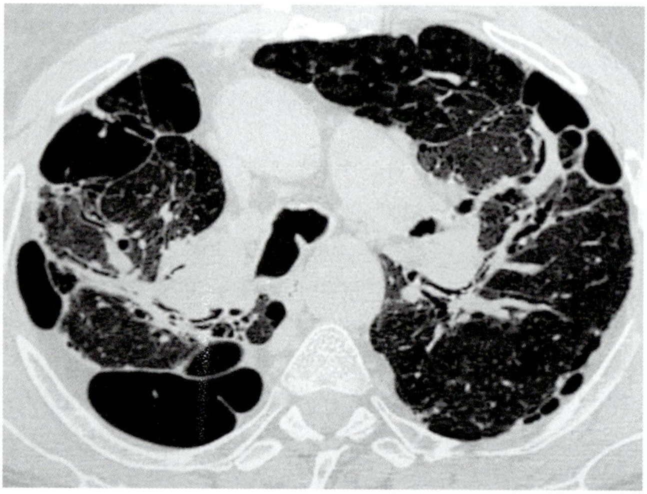

Figure 5-2 Fifty-eight year old woman with end-stage sarcoidosis. Airway distortion caused by pulmonary fibrosis in patients with advanced fibrocystic sarcoidosis, large bullae may also be observed, the cause of dyspnea.

In patients with advanced fibrocystic sarcoidosis, large bullae, distortion, mycetomas, or bronchiaectasis may be observed (Figure 5-2). Patients with stage II, III, and IV of lung sarcoidosis may present with severe degree of dyspnea as a prominent symptom, although some patients with stage I of the lung disease may also state dyspnea as the most bothersome symptom of their lung disease. Pulmonary function tests (PFTs) are reliable measure of dyspnea degree. PFT impairments are

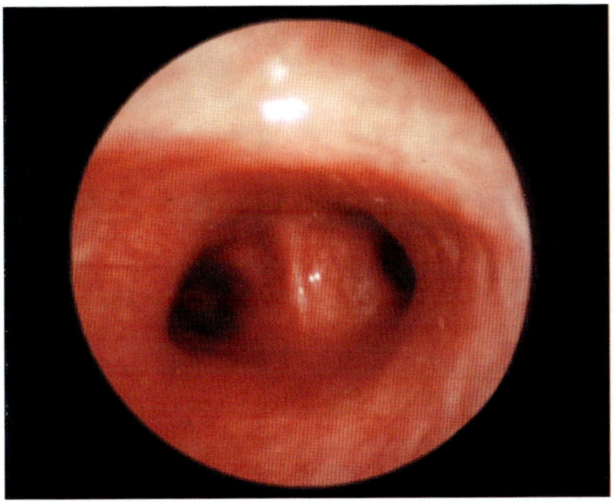

Figure 5-3 Possible cause of dyspnea in sarcoidosis. Extraluminal compression by enlarged lymph nodes narrowing the right main bronchus—endoscopic view. *Courtesy:* Professor Dragan Mandaric, Dr Emilija Bukurov-Sudjic. Department of Bronchology, Clinic of Pulmonary Diseases, Clinical Center Belgrade, Serbia.

present in 40–80% of patients with parenchymal infiltrates (stage II, III, and IV) and approximately 20% of patients with stage I of lung sarcoidosis.[25-29] Even in patients with normal chest X-ray (stage 0 of the lung disease) who present with dyspnea, forced vital capacity or diffusing capacity of the lung for carbon monoxide (DLCO) was reduced in 15–25% and 25–50%, respectively.[3,27-29]

Airway obstruction, manifested with dyspnea, with reduced forced expiratory volume in 1 second (FEV_1) and reduced expiratory flow rates was noticed in 30–50% of patients with pulmonary sarcoidosis.[29,30]

Airway obstruction in sarcoidosis may be caused by multiple facts:

- Narrowing of bronchial walls commonly due to granulomatous lesions of fibrotic traction-scarring[30,31]
- Peribronchial fibrosis[28]
- Airway distortion caused by pulmonary fibrosis[32]
- Compression by enlarged lymph nodes (Figure 5-3)[27]
- Small airways disease[15]
- Bronchial hyperreactivity.[15]

In some series, bronchial hyperreactivity has been noticed in more than 50% of the analyzed patients.[15] Computed tomography (CT) scans are useful to determine the extent and nature of stenosis in the lower respiratory tract (Figures 5-4 to 5-6).[32,33]

Lesions of the Respiratory Muscles Causing Dyspnea

Lesions of the respiratory muscles may also contribute to dyspnea in patients with sarcoidosis.[27,29] Baydur et al. measured respiratory muscle function by mouth

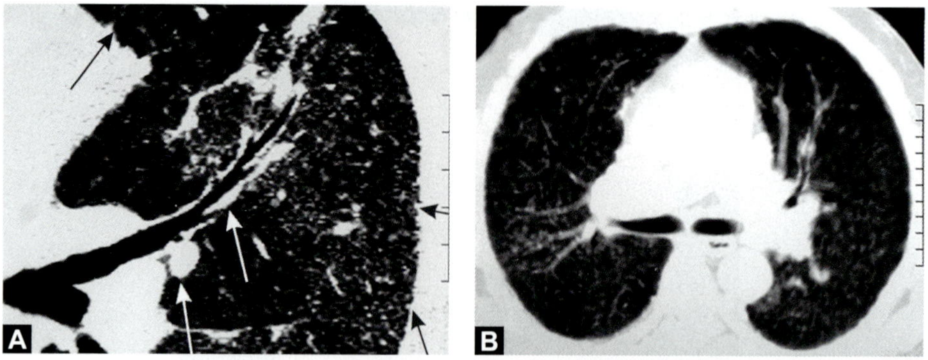

Figure 5-4 **A,** Peribronchial thickening in patient with chronic pulmonary sarcoidosis. **B,** High-resolution computed tomography scan shows extensive honeycombing, indicating irreversible fibrosis. In this patient, the diagnosis of sarcoidosis was established on open lung biopsy. Dyspnea and dry cough were predominant respiratory symptoms.

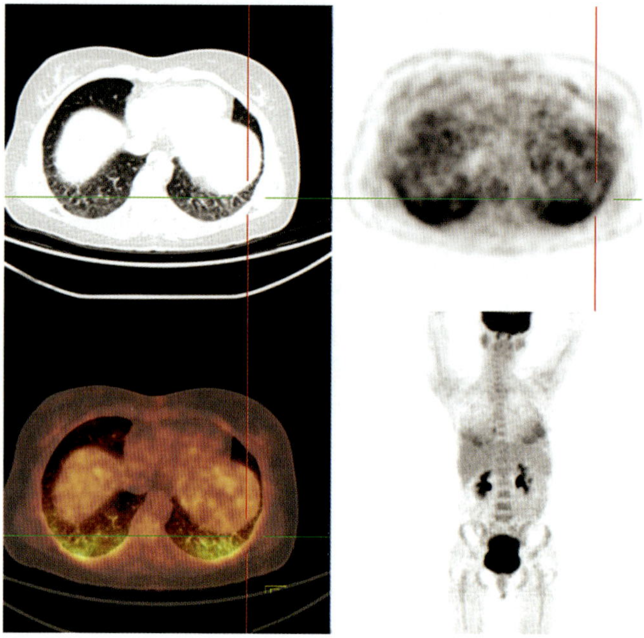

Figure 5-5 Positive pulmonary fludeoxyglucose (FDG) positron emission tomography (PET) scan findings. 18F-FDG PET scan revealing active disease, with parenchymal uptake due to sarcoidosis.

inspiratory muscle pressure and expiratory muscle pressure.[34] The authors found significant linear correlation between increasing dyspnea and decreasing respiratory muscles function in patients with sarcoidosis compared with healthy controls.[34] The interesting fact was that, in this study, the level of dyspnea did not correlate with lung volumes or DLCO.

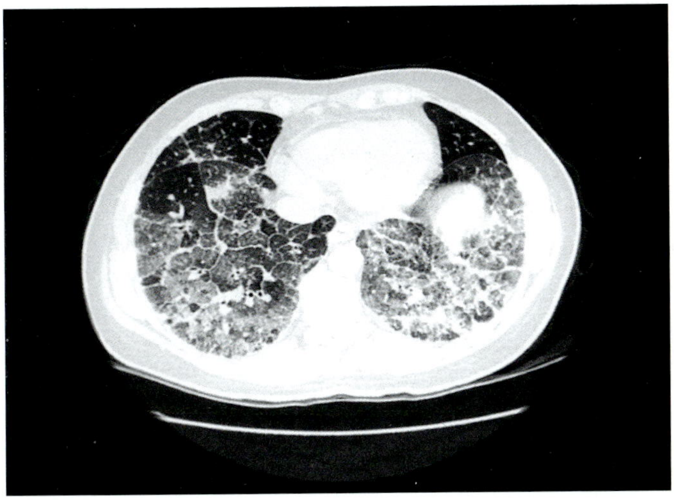

Figure 5-6 Computed tomography scan of the same patient representing areas of ground-glass attenuation (diffuse septal reticulation with distorted linear opacities). This patient had chronic sarcoidosis. The disease remitted and was not active for years. At the time, she experienced relapse the main symptom was dyspnea on exertion.

Pleural Lesions Causing Dyspnea

Pleural manifestations of sarcoidosis, i.e, pneumothorax, pleural effusion, or chylothorax that may cause clinically manifested dyspnea occur in 2–4% of patients.[35-41] The details are discussed in chapter 9 (Pleural Sarcoidosis).

Pulmonary Vascular Involvement Causing Dyspnea

Clinically manifested severe dyspnea despite the steroid therapy was reported in 50% of the analyzed patients with PAH.[17] PAH is defined as mean pulmonary arterial pressure (PAP) >25 mmHg on right heart catheterization (RHC) was present in 74% of patients in one study.[42] PFTs did not correlate with the degree of PAH.

Mechanisms responsible for PAH in sarcoidosis:

- Hypoxic vasoconstriction
- Infiltration or obliteration of pulmonary vessels by granulomatous fibrotic response (Figure 5-7)[43,44]
- Extrinsic compression of major pulmonary arteries by enlarged lymph nodes (Figure 5-8).[45]

The diagnosis of PAH may be difficult, although RHC reveals the diagnosis. The noninvasive techniques (chest CT and Doppler echocardiography) are less accurate than RHC.[46]

Patients with progressive pulmonary sarcoidosis who develop stage IV fibrocystic disease commonly manifest physiologically with varying degrees of restrictive and obstructive lung function impairments and a decreased DLCO. PAH is a recognized

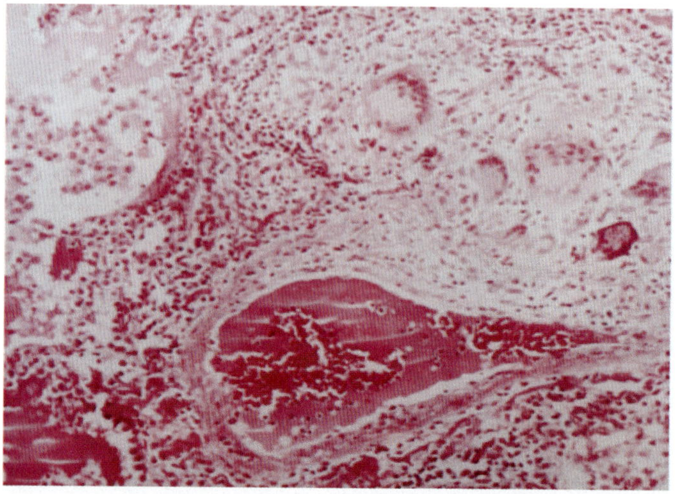

Figure 5-7 This slide demonstrates the granulomas compressing the blood vessel. This perhaps explains the severity of diffusing capacity impairment in some patients with sarcoidosis.

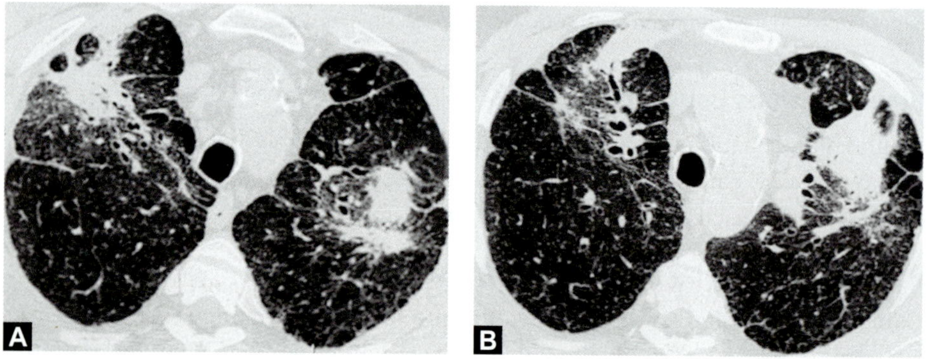

Figure 5-8 Computed tomography images. **A,** CT scan of the chest showing stage IV sarcoidosis with associated pulmonary hypertension. **B,** An enlarged pulmonary artery and fibrocystic sarcoidosis.

complication of sarcoidosis with a reported prevalence between 1 and 28% of all patients at rest and up to 43% with exercise.[47-49] PAH usually occurs in patients with stage IV of the lung disease.

Miscellaneous Lesions of the Airways Causing Dyspnea

Lesions of the Upper Respiratory Tract and Laryngeal Sarcoidosis

The upper airways including nasal and/or oral passages and larynx have been considered rare locations of sarcoidosis lesions. However, in a study of James et al., out of 818 patients with multisystem sarcoidosis, the upper respiratory tract was involved in 53 patients (6%), with the majority of 36 patients having nasal mucosal involvement.[50]

Nodular sarcoid lesions localized in supraglottic or glottic area can lead to severe dyspnea and stridor, sometimes accompanied with dysphonia and chronic cough. Endoscopy (rhinopharyngeal-laryngeal) reveals granulomatous nodular lesions.[51]

Laryngeal sarcoidosis is a phenomenon usually misdiagnosed with asthma. Sometimes it might be a cause of life-threatening occlusion of the airway.[52] However unless correct biopsy specimens are obtained, the diagnosis can be missed because the occurrence of laryngeal sarcoidosis is uncommon.[8]

REFERENCES

1. Available from: http://www.brainyquote.com/quotes/authors/s/sophocles.html
2. Harrison BD, Shaylor JM, Stokes TC, Wilkes AR. Airflow limitation in sarcoidosis--a study of pulmonary function in 107 patients with newly diagnosed disease. *Respir Med.* 1991;85:59-64.
3. Sharma OP, Johnson R. Airway obstruction in sarcoidosis. A study of 123 nonsmoking black American patients with sarcoidosis. *Chest.* 1988;94:343–6.
4. Hunninghake GW, Costabel U, Ando M, Baughman R, Cordier JF, du Bois R, et al. ATS/ERS/WASOG statement on sarcoidosis. American Thoracic Society/European Respiratory Society/World Association of Sarcoidosis and other Granulomatous Disorders. *Sarcoidosis Vasc Diffuse Lung Dis.* 1999;16:149-73.
5. Yamamoto M, Sharma OP, Hosoda Y. Special report: the 1991 descriptive definition of sarcoidosis. *Sarcoidosis.* 1992;9:33-34.
6. Davies CW, Tasker AD, Padley SP, Davies RJ, Gleeson FV. Air trapping in sarcoidosis on computed tomography: correlation with lung function. *Clin Radiol.* 2000;55:217-21.
7. Miller A, Brown LK, Teirstein AS. Stenosis of main bronchi mimicking fixed upper airway obstruction in sarcoidosis. *Chest.* 1985;88:244-8.
8. Polychronopoulos VS, Prakash UB. Airway involvement in sarcoidosis. *Chest.* 2009;136; 1371-80.
9. Westcott JL, Noehren TH. Bronchial stenosis in chronic sarcoidosis. *Chest.* 1973;63:893-7.
10. Lefrak S, Di Benedetto R. Systematic sarcoidosis with severe involvement of the upper respiratory tract. *Am Rev Respir Dis.* 1970;102:801-7.
11. Murray ME, Stokes TC. Endobronchial sarcoidosis presenting as severe upper airways narrowing with normal chest radiograph. *Respir Med.* 1991;85:425-6.
12. Akira M, Kozuka T, Inoue Y, Sakatani M. Long-term follow-up CT scan evaluation in patients with pulmonary sarcoidosis. *Chest.* 2005;127:185-91.
13. Abehsera M, Valeyre D, Grenier P, Jaillet H, Battesti JP, Brauner MW. Sarcoidosis with pulmonary fibrosis: CT patterns and correlation with pulmonary function. *AJR Am J Roentgenol.* 2000;174:1751-7.
14. Shorr AF, Torrington KG, Hnatiuk OW. Endobronchial involvement and airway hyperreactivity in patients with sarcoidosis. *Chest.* 2001;120:881-6.
15. Mihailovic-Vucinic V, Zugic V, Videnovic-Ivanov J. New observations on pulmonary function changes in sarcoidosis. *Curr Opin Pulm Med.* 2003;9:436-41.
16. Turner GA, Lower EE, Corser BC, Gunther KL, Baughman RP. Sleep apnea in sarcoidosis. *Sarcoidosis Vasc Diffuse Lung Dis.* 1997;14:61-4.
17. Baughman RB, Engel PJ, Meyer CA, Barrett AB, Lower EE. Pulmonary hypertension in sarcoidosis. *Sarcoidosis Vasc Diffuse Lung Dis.* 2006;23;108-116.
18. Chapman JT, Mehta AC. Bronchoscopy in sarcoidosis: diagnostic and therapeutic interventions. *Curr Opin Pulm Med.* 2003;9:402-7.

19. Judson MA, Strange C. Bullous sarcoidosis: a report of three cases. *Chest.* 1998;114:1474-8.
20. Gibson GJ, Prescott RJ, Muers MF, Middleton WG, Mitchell DN, Connolly CK, et al. British Thoracic Society sarcoidosis study: effects of long term corticosteroid treatment. *Thorax.* 1996;51:238-47.
21. Miller A, Teirstein AS, Jackler I, Chuang M, Siltzbach LE. Airway function in chronic pulmonary sarcoidosis with fibrosis. *Am Rev Respir Dis.* 1974;109:179-89.
22. Swigris JJ, Olson AL, Huie TJ, Fernandez-Perez ER, Solomon J, Sprunger D, et al. Sarcoidosis-related mortality in the United States from 1988 to 2007. *Am J Respir Crit Care Med.* 2011;183:1524-30.
23. Hennebicque AS, Nunes H, Brillet PY, Moulahi H, Valeyre D, Brauner MW. CT findings in severe thoracic sarcoidosis. *Eur Radiol.* 2005;15:23-30.
24. Lynch JP 3rd. Computed tomographic scanning in sarcoidosis. *Semin Respir Crit Care Med.* 2003;24:393-418.
25. Israel HL, Lenchner GS, Atkinson GW. Sarcoidosis and aspergilloma: the role of surgery. *Chest.* 1982;82:430-2.
26. Lewis MM, Mortelliti MP, Yeager H Jr, Tsou E. Clinical bronchiectasis complicating pulmonary sarcoidosis: case series of seven patients. *Sarcoidosis Vasc Diffuse Lung Dis.* 2002;19:154-9.
27. Lynch, JP 3rd, Ma YL, Koss MN, White ES. Pulmonary sarcoidosis. *Semin Respir Crit Care Med.* 2007;28:53-74.
28. Alhamad EH, Lynch JP 3rd, Martinez FJ. Pulmonary function tests in interstitial lung disease: what role do they have? *Clin Chest Med.* 2001;22:715-750, ix.
29. Subramanian I, Flaherty K, Martinez F. Pulmonary function testing in sarcoidosis. In: Baughman RP, editor. Sarcoidosis. New York: Taylor and Francis Group; 2006. p. 415-33.
30. Benatar SR, Clark TJ. Pulmonary function in a case of endobronchial sarcoidosis. *Am Rev Respir Dis.* 1974;110:490-6.
31. Chambellan A, Turbie P, Nunes H, Brauner M, Battesti JP, Valeyre D. Endoluminal stenosis of proximal bronchi in sarcoidosis: bronchoscopy, function, and evolution. *Chest.* 2005;127:472-81.
32. Miller A, Brown LK, Sloane MF, Bhuptani A, Teirstein AS. Cardiorespiratory responses to incremental exercise in sarcoidosis patients with normal spirometry. *Chest.* 1995;107: 323-9.
33. Criado E, Sánchez M, Ramírez J, Arguis P, de Caralt TM, Perea RJ, et al. Pulmonary sarcoidosis: typical and atypical manifestations at high-resolution CT with pathologic correlation. *Radiographics.* 2010;30:1567-86.
34. Baydur A, Alsalek M, Louie SG, Sharma OP. Respiratory muscle strength, lung function, and dyspnea in patients with sarcoidosis. *Chest.* 2001;120:102-8.
35. Soskel NT, Sharma OP. Pleural involvement in sarcoidosis. *Curr Opin Pulm Med.* 2000; 6:455-68.
36. Nicholls AJ, Friend JA, Legge JS. Sarcoid pleural effusion: three cases and review of the literature. *Thorax.* 1980;35:277-281.
37. Sharma OP, Gordonson J. Pleural effusion in sarcoidosis: a report of six cases. *Thorax.* 1975;30:95-101.
38. Balasubramanian P, Mathew J, Cherian R, Abraham OC. Bilateral massive pleural effusion: a rare presentation of sarcoidosis. *J Postgrad Med.* 2005;51:335-6.
39. Heidecker JT, Judson MA. Pleural effusion caused by trapped lung. *South Med J.* 2003; 96:510-1.
40. Froudarakis ME, Bouros D, Voloudaki A, Papiris S, Kottakis Y, Constantopoulos SH, et al. Pneumothorax as a first manifestation of sarcoidosis. *Chest.* 1997;112:278-80.

41. Akelsson IG, Eklund A, Skold CM, Tornling G. Bilateral spontaneous pneumothorax and sarcoidosis. *Sarcoidosis.* 1990;7:136-8.
42. Shorr AF, Helman DL, Davies DB, Nathan SD. Pulmonary hypertension in advanced sarcoidosis: epidemiology and clinical characteristics. *Eur Respir J.* 2005;25:783-8.
43. Preston IR, Klinger JR, Landzberg MJ, Houtchens J, Nelson D, Hill NS. Vasoresponsiveness of sarcoidosis-associated pulmonary hypertension. *Chest.* 2001;120:866-72.
44. Damuth TE, Bower JS, Cho K, Dantzker DR. Major pulmonary artery stenosis causing pulmonary hypertension in sarcoidosis. *Chest.* 1980;78:888-91.
45. Nunes H, Humbert M, Capron F, Brauner M, Sitbon O, Battesti JP, et al. Pulmonary hypertension associated with sarcoidosis: mechanisms, haemodynamics and prognosis. *Thorax.* 2006;61:68-74.
46. Arcasoy SM, Christie JD, Pochettino A, Rosengard BR, Blumenthal NP, Bavaria JE, et al. Characteristics and outcomes of patients with sarcoidosis listed for lung transplantation. *Chest.* 2001;120:873-80.
47. Sulica R, Teirstein AS, Kakarla S, Nemani N, Behnegar A, Padilla ML. Distinctive clinical, radiographic and functional characteristics of patients with sarcoidosis-related pulmonary hypertension. *Chest.* 2005;128:1483-9.
48. Handa T, Nagai S, Miki S, Fushimi Y, Ohta K, Mishima M, et al. Incidence of pulmonary hypertension and its clinical relevance in patients with sarcoidosis. *Chest.* 2006;129: 1246-52.
49. Oksana A, Nathan DS, Nathan DS. Management of end-stage sarcoidosis: pulmonary hypertension and lung transplantation. *Eur Respir J.* 2012;39:1520-33.
50. James DG, Barter S, Jash D, MacKinnon DM, Carstairs LS. Sarcoidosis of the upper respiratory tract (SURT). *J Laryngol Otol.* 1982;96:711-8.
51. Braun JJ, Imperiale A, Schultz P, Molard A, Charpiot A, Gentine A. Pharyngolaryngeal sarcoidosis: report of 12 cases. *Otolaryngol Head Neck Surg.* 2008;139:463-5.
52. Davis C, Girzadas DV Jr. Laryngeal sarcoidosis causing acute upper airway obstruction. *Am J Emerg Med.* 2008;26:114.e1-3.

CHAPTER

6 Chest Pain in Sarcoidosis

INTRODUCTION

Chest pain is a common symptom in many illnesses. The frequency varies and depends on the population studied. In descending order of prevalence, the following are common causes of chest pain: musculoskeletal, gastrointestinal, cardiac, psychiatric, and pulmonary. In 16% of cases, the cause remains unknown.[1]

Myocardial infarction, aortic dissection, tension pneumothorax, pulmonary infarction, esophageal rupture, and acute abdomen are some of the potentially life threatening causes.[1] In sarcoidosis, the pain is rare, but when present, is related either to enlarged hilar, mediastinal, and pericardial lymph nodes, or to left ventricular aneurysm, or both.

CLINICAL FEATURES

Nonspecific chest pain is not uncommon in sarcoidosis. In a study of 821 sarcoidosis subjects, 19% had chest pain.[2] The nature of chest pain is not explained. Smedema et al. correlated chest pain with radiological stage of the disease and found no relationship.[3] Hendricks et al., on the other hand, contended that that the enlarged hilar nodes could cause chest pain not too dissimilar from that of coronary disease.[4] The pain described with sarcoidosis can be substernal, intracapsular, or pleuritic in nature.

Curiously, enlarged nodes due to lymphoma can cause not only pain, but pain may also worsen after drinking a few glasses of alcohol. This interesting sign is called Hoster sign.[5] It has also been reported in sarcoidosis more than 30 years ago.[6] Ventricular aneurysm is a rare cause of chest pain.[7]

Occasionally, chest pain can be associated with abdominal pain. When it occurs, it is attributed to pancreatitis due to hypercalcemia and enlarged liver and spleen. In peritoneal sarcoidosis, omental involvement and diffuse adenopathy most likely accounts for the abdominal pain. A laparoscopic peritoneal-omental biopsy can reveal noncaseating granulomas.[8]

TREATMENT

A short course of prednisone 40 mg daily over a period of 4–6 weeks ameliorates the pain.

CASE STUDY

A 52-year old African-American woman presented to emergency room with a history of substernal pain of 1 week duration. The pain was intermittent, did not radiate preferentially, and was not affected by exercise or change in position. On examination, she had normal vital signs. Multiple 2 × 2 nontender movable lymph nodes in the anterior, posterior, and submandibular areas were present. Examination of the lungs, heart, eyes, skin, and joints was normal.

Laboratory analysis revealed mild anemia. Metabolic panel, liver function tests, serum calcium, and serum angiotensin levels were normal. Urine examination showed no red cells. An electrocardiogram showed normal sinus rhythm without ST-T wave changes. Serial troponin levels were normal. A chest X-ray film showed bilateral hilar and mediastinal adenopathy with no parenchymal infiltrate. A CT of the chest and abdomen showed thoracic, pericardial, peripancreatic, and omental lymph glands (Figure 6-1). A coronary angiogram showed a preserved ventricular function, normal coronary arteries, and a ventricular aneurysm. Position emission tomography (PET) revealed diffuse uptake of 18-fluorodeoxyglucose by enlarged thoracic and abdominal lymph nodes (Figure 6-2). A mediastinal lymph node biopsy showed noncaseating granulomas (Figure 6-3). Acid fast bacilli and fungal tests were negative. She was given prednisone 40 mg a day. Over the course of a few months, her symptoms subsided. Serial computed tomography scans showed reduced size of the multiple lymph nodes. After 4 years, she remains asymptomatic.

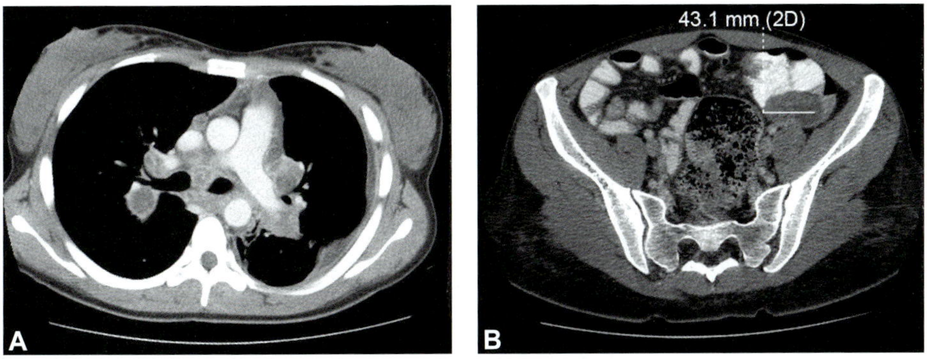

Figure 6-1A and B The chest and abdominal computed tomography presenting multiple enlarged lymph nodes (both mediastinal and abdominal). Final diagnostic procedure (biopsy) revealed noncaseating granulomas compatible with sarcoidosis.

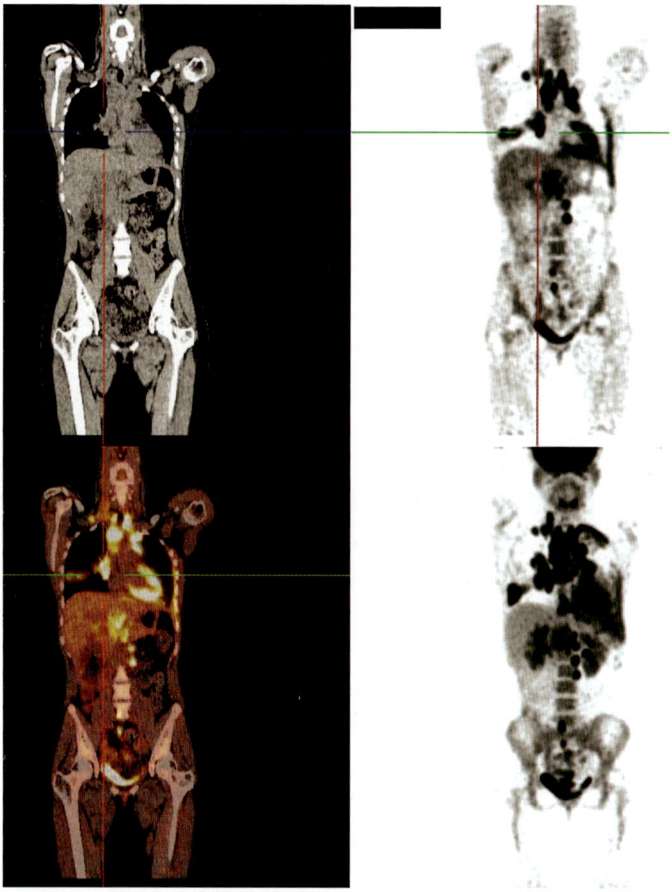

Figure 6-2 Positron emission tomography scans of the same patient also revealed diffuse uptake of 18 fluorodeoxyglucose by enlarged lymph nodes both thoracic and abdominal.

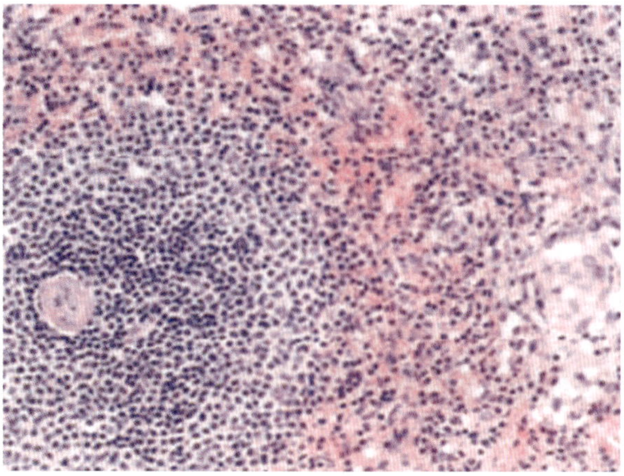

Figure 6-3 Noncaseating granuloma of the lymph node.

REFERENCES

1. Klinkman MS, Stevens D, Gorenflo DW. Episodes of care for chest pain: a preliminary report from MIRNET. Michigan Research Network. *J Fam Pract.* 1994;38:345-52.
2. Hoitsma E, De Vries J, van Santen-Hoeufft M, Faber CG, Drent M. Impact of pain in a Dutch sarcoidosis patient population. *Sarcoidosis Vasc Diffuse Lung Dis.* 2003;20:33-9.
3. Smedema J, Snoep G, van Kroonenburgh MP, van Geuns RJ, Dassen WR, Gorgels AP, et al. Cardiac involvement in patients with pulmonary sarcoidosis assessed in two university centers in Netherland. *Chest.* 2005;128:30-5.
4. Hendrick D, Blackwood R, Black J. Chest pain in the presentation of sarcoidosis. *Br J Dis Chest.* 1976;70:206-10.
5. Hoster HA. Hodgkin's disease. *Am J Roentgenol Radium Ther.* 1950;64:913-8.
6. Sharma O, Balchum O. Alcohol-induced pain and itching on hot shower in sarcoidosis. An unusual association. *Am Rev Respir Dis.* 1972;106:763-6.
7. Toda G, Iliev I, Kawahara F, Hayano M, Yano K. Left ventricular aneurysm without coronary artery disease: incidence and clinical features, analysis of 11 cases. *Intern Med.* 2000;39:531-6.
8. Gupta D, Agarwal R, Singh A, Joshi K. A "respiratory" cause o abdominal pain. *Eur Respir J.* 2006;27:430-3.

CHAPTER

7 Red Eye

DEFINITION

Red eye is a nonspecific term to describe an eye that is red or pink due to hyperemia of the superficial blood vessels of the conjunctiva, sclera, and episclera. As these structures can be affected by sarcoidosis, it becomes an important cause of a red eye. The redness or pinkish hue may or may not be associated with photophobia, gritty sensation, and watery discharge.

INCIDENCE

Ocular changes occur in about one-quarter of the patients with sarcoidosis, but the incidence varies considerably, depending on racial composition of the series and whether a thorough eye examination, including a slit examination was performed. In Japan, more than half of the patients with sarcoidosis have ocular involvement. In Europe, about one-third of the patients may be affected.[1] Ocular sarcoidosis is more common in patients with human leukocyte antigen polymorphism DRB1*1101, suggesting a genetic basis.[2]

LESIONS OF OCULAR SARCOIDOSIS

Acute granulomatous uveitis is the most common of all ocular lesions of sarcoidosis—it can be acute or chronic (Figure 7-1). Of the 442 patients studied by James et al., 89 (22%) had uveitis as a presenting feature.[3] Thirty-nine of Scadding's 275 patients had uveitis at some stage of their disease.[4] Crick et al. performed a through eye examination on 185 patients, 61 (33%) had evidence of uveitis.[5]

Subacute uveitis or iridocyclitis presents with watering and redness of eyes, cloudy vision, and photophobia. Circumcorneal ciliary injection is present, pupils are irregular, and "mutton fat" keratic precipitates are prominent in the anterior chamber. The aqueous humor may be turbid. Nodules on the iris occur rarely.

Chronic uveitis develops slowly and may lead to adhesions between the iris and the lens, glaucoma, cataract formation, and blindness. Ciliary congestion is absent.

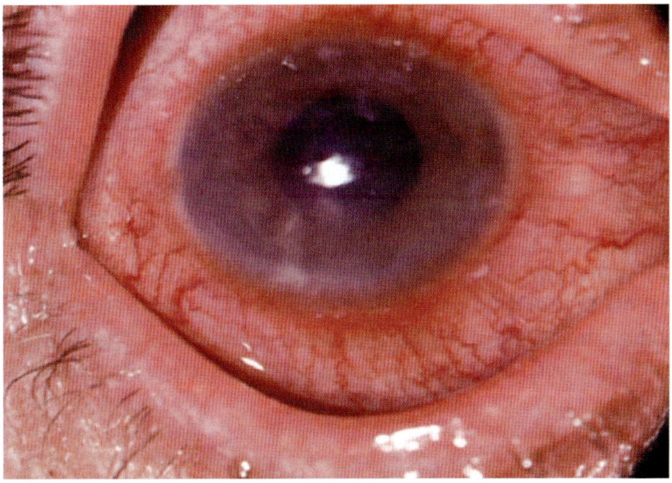

Figure 7-1 Red eye in sarcoidosis. Acute granulomatous uveitis—the most common of all ocular lesions of sarcoidosis.

The patient usually complains diminished visual and blurry vision. Posterior uveitis is much more common than is realized. Evidence of posterior uveitis was present in 44 (66%) of 61 patients in a study by Crick et al. and in 11 (25%) of patients in a study by James et al. 42 patients. Examination of fundi may reveal choroidal waxy nodules, peripheral phlebitis, retinal edema, and retinal detachment.

Conjunctival follicles are tiny, translucent, pale yellow nodules occurring in the fornices, palpebral conjunctiva, and occasionally on the bulbar conjunctiva. Crick et al. observed conjunctival follicles in 79 (56 %) of 139 patients. In 20 of these, biopsies revealed noncaseating granulomas.[6]

Conjunctivitis occurred in 14 (3%) of the patients in one series; 8 of these had erythema nodosum and bilateral hilar adenopathy. The lesion is usually bilateral.[7]

DIFFERENTIAL DIAGNOSIS

There are 3 important symptoms in a red eye: reduced visual acuity, severe ocular pain, and photophobia (light sensitivity). The presence of photophobia suggests corneal injury. "Grittiness" and foreign body sensation is almost always present in corneal injury. Bacterial keratitis may or may not affect vision but typically causes photophobia and foreign body sensation. A patient with reduced vision should be immediately seen by an ophthalmologist. Bacterial conjunctivitis is typically not associated with reduction in visual acuity, foreign body sensation, or photophobia. Morning crusting and watery discharge may be caused by allergic or viral conjunctivitis or a sty. Bacterial conjunctivitis of bacterial keratitis may cause opaque discharge.

Conjunctivitis (allergic or viral) and subconjunctival hemorrhage are the two most common cause of red eye in clinical practice. Others include blepharitis, acute glaucoma, keratitis, episcleritis, iritis, and dry eye syndrome (Table 7-1).

DIAGNOSTIC APPROACH

Diagnosis of ocular sarcoidosis is relatively easy if the typical eye lesions, including the granulomatous uveitis, conjunctival follicles, and lacrimal gland enlargement are associated with erythema nodosum, bilateral hilar and peripheral lymphadenopathy, and high angiotensin converting enzyme level in serum or tears. When the eye lesions occur in the absence of clinical features of sarcoidosis, conjunctival and lacrimal biopsies are required to demonstrate noncaseating granulomas. The sarcoidologist conducting an eye examination should be attentive to the warning symptoms of blurry vision, severe pain, photophobia, colored halos, and reduced visual activity. Clinical signs of ciliary flush, corneal opacification, corneal ulcer, pupillary abnormalities, shallow anterior chamber, and proptosis require special attention.

TREATMENT

Anterior uveitis responds to topical glucorticosteroids. Prednisolone acetate 1% drops with a dilating drops, such as scopolamine (0.25%) or cyclo-pentolate (1%) can relieve the pain due spasm of the muscle controlling the pupil and also prevent the formation of posterior synechiae. Posterior uveitis generally requires systemic corticosteroids. The use of cytotoxic and anticytokine drugs is still under investigation.

PROGNOSIS

Ocular sarcoidosis is a serious debilitating complication of sarcoidosis. All patients should have an initial complete eye-examination by an ophthalmologist. Untreated sarcoidosis can cause cataracts, glaucoma, and even blindness.

Table 7-1 Causes of "Red Eye"

Systemic inflammation	*Infectious*	*Miscellaneous*
Sarcoidosis	Toxoplasmosis	Cannabis use
Idiopathic panuveitis	HIV/CMV	High stress
Spondyloarthropathy	Tuberculosis	Rocky Mountain spotted fever
Systemic lupus erythematosis	Histoplasmosis	Trauma
Wegener's granulomatosis	Lyme disease	Parasites
Relapsing polychondritis	Syphilis	
Behcet's disease	Herpes simplex virus	

HIV, human immunodeficiency virus; CMV, cytomegalovirus.

REFERENCES

1. Ohara K, Judson M, Baughman R. Clinical aspects of ocular sarcoidosis. *Eur Respir Mon.* 2005;32:188-209.
2. Rossman M, Thompson B, Frederick M, Maliarik M, Iannuzzi MC, Rybicki BA, et al. HLA-DRB1*1101: a significant risk factor for sarcoidosis in blacks and whites. *Am J Hum Genet.* 2003;73:720-35.
3. James D, Anderson R, Langley D, Ainslie D. Ocular sarcoidosis. *Br J Ophthalmol.* 1964; 48:461-70.
4. Scadding J. Sarcoidosis. London: Eyre and Spottiswoode; 1964.
5. Crick RP, Hoyle C, Smellie H. The eyes in sarcoidosis. *Br J Ophthalmol.* 1961;5:461-81.
6. Crick R, Hoyle C, Mather G. Conjunctival biopsy in sarcoidosis. *Br Med J.* 1955;2:1180-1.
7. Karma A. Ophthalmic changes in sarcoidosis. *Acta Ophthalmol Suppl.* 1977:1-94.

CHAPTER

8 Hemoptysis in Sarcoidosis

DEFINITION

Hemoptysis is expectoration of blood with coughing. It is a manifestation of many different pulmonary problems. The symptom is frightening and can be life-threatening.

CAUSES

There are many causes of hemoptysis (Table 8-1). The pulmonary causes of hemoptysis include tuberculosis, bronchiectasis, cystic fibrosis, pulmonary embolus, and lung cancer. The common cardiac cause is mitral stenosis. Infrequently, pulmonary vasculitis, arteriovenous malformation, aortic aneurysm, and sarcoidosis can cause hemoptysis. The presence of associated symptoms helps to form a differential diagnosis. Sputum production when purulent indicates an infectious cause of hemoptysis. Weight loss and chronic cough in a patient with hemoptysis who smokes indicate malignancy. In tuberculosis, hemoptysis may be associated with low grade evening fever, weight loss, and night sweats. Hemoptysis with frothy pink sputum in a recumbent patient with heart diseases indicates pulmonary edema. Acute chest pain, sudden shortness of breath, and hemoptysis constitute a diagnostic triad for pulmonary infarction/embolism. Anemia, skin rashes, joint pains, fever, and uveitis may accompany hemoptysis in systemic vasculitis. Chronic fibrotic sarcoidosis with fungus ball can rarely cause fatal hemoptysis.

SEVERITY OF HEMOPTYSIS

Massive hemoptysis is generally greater than 600 mL in 24 hours. It can be fatal if not managed promptly. More commonly, patients with hemoptysis have lesser

Table 8-1 Some Common Cause of Hemoptysis

• Bronchiectasis	• Aspergilloma (sarcoidosis, cystic fibrosis)
• Tuberculosis	• Necrotizing pneumonia
• Bronchogenic carcinoma	• Arteriovenous malformation
• Pulmonary embolism/infarction	• Vasculitis/bleeding diathesis

quantities of blood described as specks, streaks, or clots. A tickle, rustle, or fullness in the chest can occasionally localize the side from which the blood is coming. In a patient with massive hemoptysis, the initial steps are to correctly position the patient, establish a patent airway, ensure adequate gas exchange and cardiovascular function, and control the bleeding. The source of bleeding may be identified either during efforts to control the bleeding or during a careful evaluation after the patient has been stabilized.

ASPERGILLOMA AND HEMOPTYSIS IN SARCOIDOSIS

Aspergillomas arise in preexisting pulmonary cavities due to tuberculosis, sarcoidosis, chronic obstructive pulmonary disease, and necrotizing pneumonias that have become colonized with aspergillus organisms.[1] Aspergilloma or a fungus ball, composed of *Aspergillus hyphae*, fibrin, mucus, and cellular debris is not uncommon in sarcoidosis, particularly in patients with cystic parenchymal damage (Figure 8-1). Many patients remain asymptomatic and stable over months and years. However, progression to chronic cavitary pulmonary aspergillosis, sometimes with extensive fibrosis, is common and can occur silently, so continued observation is required.[2,3] Spontaneous resolution of the aspergilloma occurs in fewer than 10% of patients. Wollschlager and Khan[4] reported their 10-year observation of 100 histologically-proven sarcoidosis patients for the development of aspergillomas. Serum precipitins against *Aspergillus* antigens were used to screen

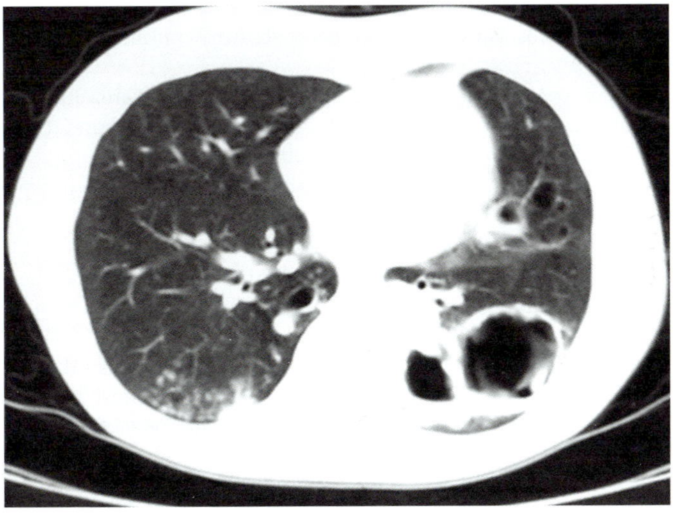

Figure 8-1 Patient with chronic progressive form of lung sarcoidosis stage III/IV and aspergilloma. Computed tomography represents almost destroyed lung parenchyma with cystic formations. Patient has massive hemoptysis the reason of frequent hospitalizations.

all patients. Twelve patients had serum precipitins and were further investigated with tomography and serial serum precipitins testing. Ten of these 12 patients had aspergillomas and 2 patients died of massive hemoptysis. No aspergillomas occurred in stages I, II, or noncystic stage III patients. All 10 aspergillomas developed in the 19 stage III patients with cystic parenchymal damage.[4]

MANAGEMENT

There is no standardized therapy for aspergilloma. Surgery is the treatment of choice for symptomatic aspergilloma, but it is also associated with high mortality and morbidity. Surgical resection offered to prevent or treat potentially life-threatening hemoptysis is usually curative, particularly in the patients with good respiratory functions.[5] Recurrent infections, inability to take azole therapy, azole resistance, and suspected malignancy are additional indications for surgical resection.[2]

When surgery is not feasible, itraconazole is the drug commonly used for the medical treatment of aspergilloma. A long-term therapy can be associated with the development of itraconazole resistance. Susceptibility testing of strains is of value to detect resistance. In these patients, voriconazole is a good alternative drug.[6] Voriconazole can be given by mouth and has a good *in vitro* activity against most of the itraconazole-resistant strains of *A. fumigatus*.[7]

REFERENCES

1. Smith NL, Denning DW. Underlying conditions in chronic pulmonary aspergillosis including simple aspergilloma. *Eur Resp J.* 2011;37:865-72.
2. Soubani AO, Chandrasekar PH. The clinical spectrum of pulmonary aspergillosis. *Chest.* 2002;121:1988-99.
3. Criado E, Sánchez M, Ramírez J, Arguis P, de Caralt TM, Perea RJ, et al. Pulmonary sarcoidosis: typical and atypical manifestations at high-resolution CT correlation with pathologic correlation. *Radiographics.* 2010;30:1567-86.
4. Wollschlager C, Khan F. Aspergillomas complicating sarcoidosis. A prospective study in 100 patients. *Chest.* 1984;86:585-8.
5. Israel HL, Ostrow A. Sarcoidosis and aspergilloma. *Am J Med.* 1969;47:243-50.
6. Kravitz JN, Steed LL, Judson MA. Intracavitary voriconazole for the treatment of hemoptysis complicating Pseudallescheria angusta pulmonary mycetomas in fibrocystic sarcoidosis. *Med Mycol.* 2011;49:198-201.
7. Dannaoui E, Garcia-Hermoso D, Naccache JM, Meneau I, Sanglard D, Bouges-Michel C, et al. Use of voriconazole in a patient with aspergilloma caused by an itraconazole-resistant strain of Aspergillus fumigatus. *J Med Microbiol.* 2006;55:1457-9.

CHAPTER

9 Sarcoidosis of the Pleura

HISTORY

Since the first report by Schaumann on pleural sarcoidosis in 1933, pleural involvement remained a rare manifestation of sarcoidosis in all published series.[1]

INCIDENCE

The overall prevalence of pleural sarcoidosis is difficult to evaluate because of incomplete reporting. The usage of computed tomographic (CT) scans, especially high resolution CT (HRCT) has increased the awareness of this manifestation of sarcoidosis, allowing detection of delicate cases of pleural sarcoid involvement. In a large study of Kostina et al.,[2] out of 2,775 analyzed pulmonary sarcoidosis cases, 278 (10%) had some form of pleural manifestation. The precise incidence of pleural sarcoidosis varies from 0.7% to almost 10%.[3-8]

CLINICAL MANIFESTATIONS

Types of pleural involvement in sarcoidosis include:

- Pleural effusion
- Hemothorax
- Pleural thickening
- Chylothorax
- Pneumothorax
- Pleural nodules.

All types of pleural involvement in sarcoidosis have predominant location on the right side (52.7%), however, the explanation remains unclear. In a majority of cases, pleural involvement occurs mainly in the later stages of the disease.[8]

Earlier reports noted that pleural involvement in sarcoidosis was typically associated with widespread parenchymal lung disease.[5,9]

DIAGNOSIS

HRCT scanning can detect micronodules lining the visceral pleural surface, pleural thickening, pleural effusion, or pneumothorax. It is mandatory to carefully evaluate histologically all types of pleural involvement, because of the possibility of pleural tuberculosis or mesothelioma.[8,10]

PLEURAL EFFUSION

The precise data on the incidence of pleural effusion as a manifestation of pleural sarcoidosis varies. A large series by Kostina et al. detected only 3 pleural effusions (Figures 9-1 and 9-2) among 2,775 patients with pulmonary sarcoidosis.[2] The incidence also depends on the sensitivity of the diagnostic procedures and is more common when more sensitive tests are used. In a recent prospective study, thoracic ultrasonograms were performed in 181 consecutive outpatients with sarcoidosis. Pleural effusions were detected in 5 (2.8%) but only 3 were attributed to sarcoidosis, 2 were a manifestation of congestive heart failure.[11]

Most of the pleural effusions due to sarcoidosis are small or modest in size. Cases of massive pleural effusions have been described.[12] When present, sarcoid pleural effusions are usually asymptomatic.[8] In one case, pleural sarcoidosis with "trapped lung" required decortication for relief of symptoms.[13]

The appearance of pleural fluid is commonly serous, with the mean pleural fluid protein concentration of about 4.0 mg/dL.[11] Lymphocytosis with predominance of CD4 lymphocytes occurs in two-thirds of cases.[14] Eosinophilic pleural effusion is infrequent.[4,8,11,15,16]

PLEURAL THICKENING

Pleural thickening may be observed when sensitive techniques are applied but is usually not associated with clinical symptoms. One study using HRCT cited

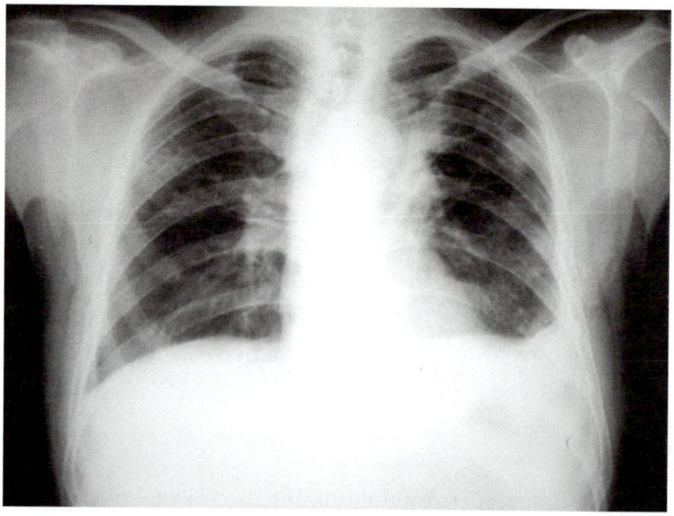

Figure 9-1 Pleural effusion in sarcoidosis on chest X-ray.

pleural thickening in 9% of sarcoid patients.[17] The incidence is higher in patients with chronic fibrocystic sarcoidosis (Figure 9-3). Tumor like infiltrations of pleural sarcoidosis not detectable at chest X-ray are rare.[18]

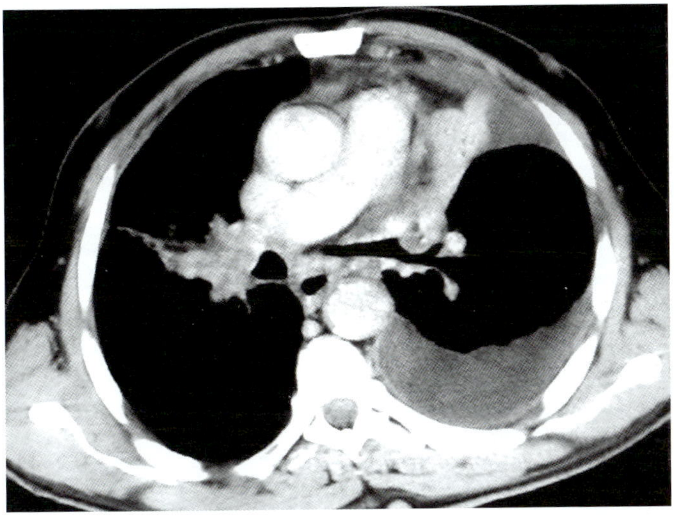

Figure 9-2 Thoracic computed tomography of a patient representing pleural effusion.

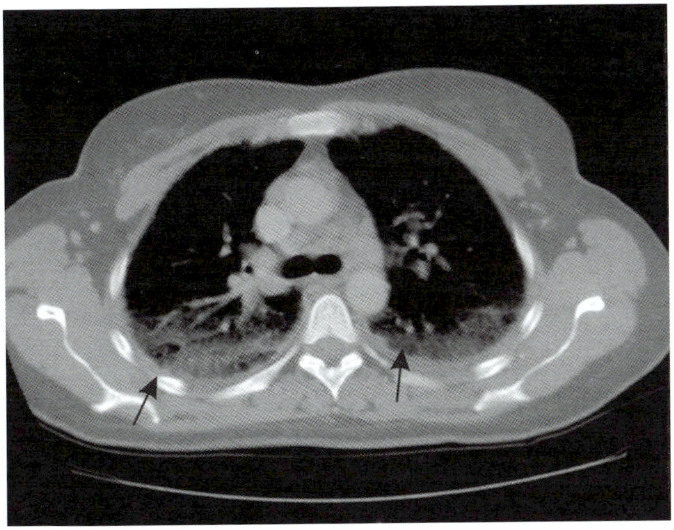

Figure 9-3 Computed tomography (CT) scan showing pleural thickening in patient with chronic sarcoidosis. The diagnosis of sarcoidosis was obtained in 2002 on bronchoscopy. This CT scan was made when the patient experienced relapse of disease. First, this patient was treated with steroids successfully. For almost 5 years, she was experiencing sarcoidosis remission without any therapy. However, a year ago her disease became active.

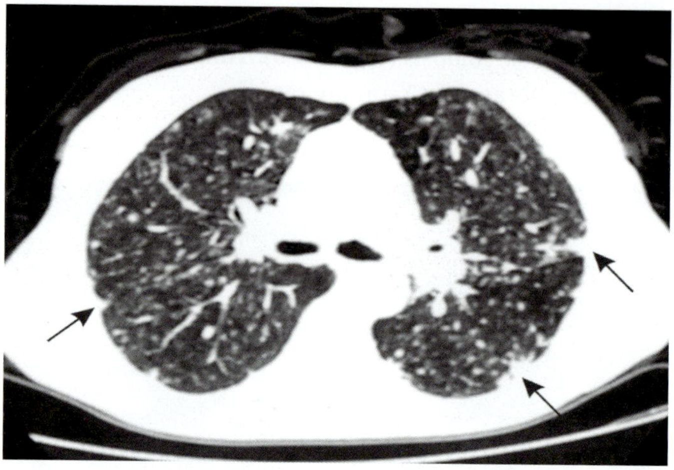

Figure 9-4 Subpleural nodules in a 72 years old patient with sarcoidosis. This may also represent sarcoidosis in the aged because this was the first onset of sarcoidosis in 8 decade of the female patient.

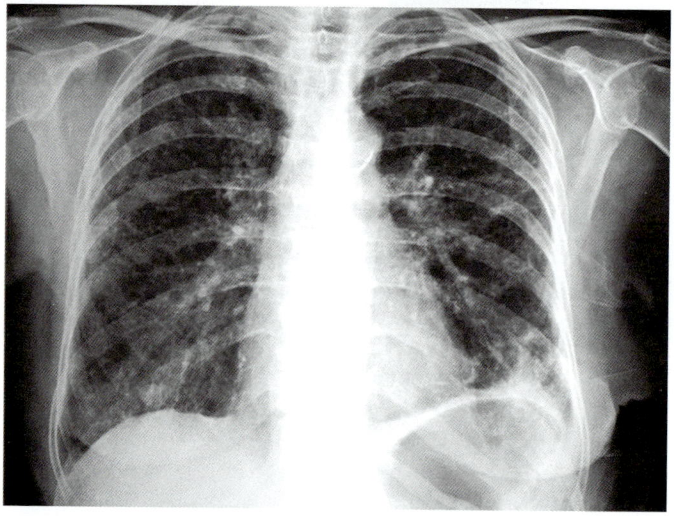

Figure 9-5 Chest X-ray of the above patient, with diffuse reticular lesions of the lung parenchyma. Open lung biopsy revealed sarcoidosis.

SUBPLEURAL NODULES

Subpleural nodules are observed by HRCT in 22–76% of sarcoidosis cases (Figure 9-4 and 9-5). They rarely cause symptoms.[10,19-21]

PNEUMOTHORAX

Pneumothorax may complicate sarcoidosis due to rupture of bullae or necrosis of subpleural granulomas (Figure 9-6).[2,8,22-26]

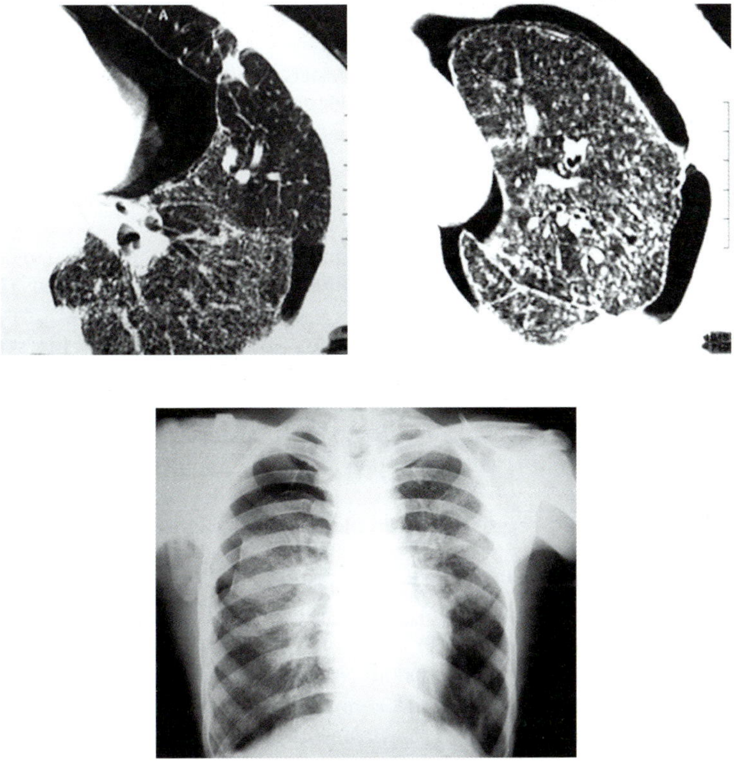

Figure 9-6 Posterioanterior chest X-ray and high resolution computed tomography representing patient with loculated pneumothorax in patient with fibrocystic sarcoidosis.

Chylothorax

Only a few cases of chylothorax have been reported.[27,28]

Hemothorax

To date, only one patient with hemothorax due to sarcoidosis has been described.[8]

REFERENCES

1. Schaumann MJ. Etude anatomo-patholgique et histologique sur les localizations vicerales de la lymphogranulomatose benigne. *Bull Soc Fr Dermatol Syphiligr.* 1933;40:1167-78.
2. Kostina ZI, Ivanovskii VB, Voloshko IV, Kol'nikova OV, Khorovskaia LA. Diagnosis and treatment of pleural lesions in sarcoidosis of the respiratory organs. *Probl Tuberk.* 1992:21-3.
3. Chusid EL, Siltzbach LE. Sarcoidosis of the pleura. *Ann Intern Med.* 1974;81:190-4.
4. Sharma OP, Gordonson J. Pleural effusion in sarcoidosis: a report of six cases. *Thorax.* 1975;30:95-101.
5. Beekman JF, Zimmet SM, Chun BK, Miranda AA, Katz S. Spectrum of pleural involvement in sarcoidosis. *Arch Intern Med.* 1976;136:323-30.

6. Wilen SB, Rabinowitz JG, Ulreich S, Lyons HA. Pleural involvement is sarcoidosis. *Am J Med.* 1974;57:200-9.
7. Tommasini A, Di Vittorio G, Facchinetti F, Festi G, Schito V, Cipriani A. Pleural effusions in sarcoidosis: a case report. *Sarcoidosis.* 1994;11:138-40.
8. Soskel NT, Sharma OP. Pleural involvement in sarcoidosis. *Curr Opin Pulm Med.* 2000; 6:455-68.
9. Ellis K, Renthal G. Pulmonary sarcoidosis: roentgenographic observations on course of disease. *AJR Am J Roentgenol.* 1962;88:1070-83.
10. Remy-Jardin M, Beuscart R, Sault MC, Marquette CH, Remy J. Subpleural micronodules in diffuse infiltrative lung diseases: evaluation with thin-section CT scans. *Radiology.* 1990;177:133-9.
11. Huggins JT, Doelken P, Sahn SA, King L, Judson MA. Pleural effusions in a series of 181 outpatients with sarcoidosis. *Chest.* 2006;129:1599-604.
12. Balasubramanian P, Mathew J, Cherian R, Abraham OC. Bilateral massive pleural effusion: a rare presentation of sarcoidosis. *J Postgrad Med.* 2005;51:335-6.
13. Heidecker JT, Judson MA. Pleural effusion caused by trapped lung. *South Med J.* 2003; 96:510-1.
14. Nicholls AJ, Friend JA, Legge JS. Sarcoid pleural effusion: three cases and review of the literature. *Thorax.* 1980;35:277-81.
15. Flammang d'Ortho MP, Cadranel J, Milleron BJ, Akoun GM. Pleural, alveolar and blood T-lymphocyte subsets in pleuro pulmonary sarcoidosis. *Chest.* 1990;98:782-3.
16. Durand DV, Dellinger A, Guerin C, Guerin JC, Levrat R. Pleural sarcoidosis: one case presenting with an eosinophilic effusion. *Thorax.* 1984;39:468-9.
17. Brauner MW, Grenier P, Mompoint D, Lenoir S, de Cremoux H. Pulmonary sarcoidosis: evaluation with highresolution CT. *Radiology.* 1989;172:467-1.
18. Bergstrom CE, Eklund A. Sarcoidosis with pleural involvement mimicking a coin lesion. *Sarcoidosis.* 1990;7:78-9.
19. Loughney E, Higgins BG. Pleural sarcoidosis: a rare presentation. *Thorax.* 1997;52:200-1.
20. Muller NL, Mawson JB, Mathieson JR, Abboud R, Ostrow DN, Champion P. Sarcoidosis: correlation of extent of disease at CT with clinical, functional, and radiographic findings. *Radiology.* 1989;171:613-8.
21. Miller BH, Rosado-de-Christenson ML, McAdams HP, Fishback NF. Thoracic sarcoidosis: radiologic-pathologic correlation. *Radiographics.* 1995;15:421-37.
22. Soskel N, Sharma OP. Pleural involvement in sarcoidosis: case presentation and detailed review of the literature. *Semin Respir Med.* 1992;13:492-514.
23. Froudarakis ME, Bouros D, Voloudaki A, Papiris S, Kottakis Y, Constantopoulos SH, et al. Pneumothorax as a first manifestation of sarcoidosis. *Chest.* 1997;112:278-80.
24. Akelsson IG, Eklund A, Skold CM, Tornling G. Bilateral spontaneous pneumothorax and sarcoidosis. *Sarcoidosis.* 1990;7:136-8.
25. Ross RJ, Empey DW. Bilateral spontaneous pneumothorax in sarcoidosis. *Postgrad Med J.* 1983;59:106-7.
26. Gomm SA. An unusual presentation of sarcoidosis: spontaneous haemopneumothorax. *Postgrad Med J.* 1984;60:621-3.
27. Jarman PR, Whyte MK, Sabroe I, Hughes JM. Sarcoidosis presenting with chylothorax. *Thorax.* 1995;50:1324-5.
28 Parker JM, Torrington KG, Phillips YY. Sarcoidosis complicated by chylothorax. *South Med J.* 1994;87:860-2.

CHAPTER

10 Erythema Nodosum and Löfgren's Syndrome

DEFINITION

Erythema nodosum (EN), a common skin hypersensitivity reaction, consists of red, tender, shining, nodules over the shins, calves, and buttocks. Fever, malaise, and polyarthralgias occur in 50% of patients having EN.

CAUSES

In the second half of the 19th century, "rheumatism" was the main cause of EN and tuberculosis the second. During the first half of the 20th century, tuberculosis was considered to be the cause of EN in over 90% of adult patients. During the second half of the 20th century, sarcoidosis, Behcet's disease, fungal infections, and drug-reactions were added to the list (Table 10-1). Oral contraceptives can occasionally trigger the reaction.

Table 10-1 Differential Diagnosis of Common Causes of Erythema Nodosum

Disease	*Clinical features*	*Skin test*	*Laboratory tests*	*Chest X-ray*
Streptococcal infection	Upper respiratory infection	None	ASO titers	Unhelpful
Tuberculosis	Asians, migrants, AIDS	Positive tuberculin test	High ESR	Unilateral hilar adenopathy, upper lobe lung infiltrate
Sarcoidosis	Scandinavians, Irish, English	Positive Kveim-Siltzbach test, negative tuberculin	Raised serum angiotensin converting enzyme	Bilateral hilar adenopathy with or without pulmonary infiltrate
Coccidioido-mycosis	San Joaquin, California (endemic area)	Positive coccidioidin test	Complement-fixation antibodies	Unilateral/ bilateral hilar adenopathy, lung infiltrate/ cavity

Continued

Continued

Histoplasmosis	Ohio, Mississippi valley delta, Mexico, Central and South America	Histoplasmin test	Complement fixation antibodies	Hilar adenopathy/ pulmonary infiltrate
Lepromatous leprosy	Tropical countries, sensory loss, iritis	Lepromin test	Skin or nerve biopsy for *M. leprae*	Not helpful
Behcet's disease	Turkey, Mediter-ranean littoral, China, Japan	Pathergy, raised Serum IgD level	Biopsy rarely helpful	Not helpful

ASO, antistreptolysin O; AIDS, acquired immunodeficiency syndrome; IgD, immunoglobulin D; ESR, erythrocyte sedimentation rate.

CLINICAL FEATURES

In 1798, Robert Willan, a British dermatologist introduced the term EN, "...many of the red patches are large and rounded. The central part of them are very gradually elevated and on the 6th or 7th day form hard and painful protuberances. From the 7th to 10th day, they constantly soften without ulceration. On the 8th and 9th day, the red color changes to bluish or livid, and the affected limb appears as if it has been severely bruised... I have only seen it in females, most of whom were servants. Irregular shivering, nausea, headaches, and fretfulness with a quick unequal pulse and whitish fur on the tongue precede it. The EN usually affects the foreparts of the legs".[1]

EN is the hallmark of acute sarcoidosis. EN associated with acute pulmonary sarcoidosis occurred in 251 (31%) of the 818 patients studied in England. It was more common in women of childbearing age, and also more frequent in the spring. EN pinpointed the onset of sarcoidosis in 640 (17%) of 3,676 patients in a worldwide sarcoidosis survey. The distribution was uneven, for it occurred in one-third of the 3 British series, London, Edinburgh, and Reading, but was less evident elsewhere. It was never a presenting feature of sarcoidosis in Tokyo. In British sarcoidosis patients (as distinct from West Indian patients), EN occurred more frequently in patients with human leukocyte antigen (HLA)-B8, HLA-A1, HLA-CW7, or HLA-DR3.

Löfgren syndrome consists of EN and bilateral hilar adenopathy on a chest X-ray film. The hilar enlargement is characteristically symmetrical, although a larger number of lymph nodes on the right side may produce an impression of pronounced right-sided enlargement. In addition to bilateral hilar enlargement, the right paratracheal adenopathy is often present.

This symmetrical enlargement of the hilar and mediastinal adenopathy differs from the asymmetrical enlargement seen in lymphoma, bronchogenic carcinoma, and metastatic malignancies. The symmetrical enlargement of hilar lymph nodes in an asymptomatic person or one with EN or iridocyclitis is rarely due to anything but sarcoidosis.

The combination of EN and bilateral hilar adenopathy predicts a favorable outcome of sarcoidosis. Löfgren reported that patients with EN and bilateral hilar adenopathy without accompanying radiographic parenchymal lesions showed a complete radiographic clearance within 2 years.[2]

PATHOLOGY

Under the microscope, EN is a septal panniculitis. In the early stages, septal infiltrate of neutrophils, with occasional eosinophils, appears in association with vascular edema. In the vicinity of connective tissue septa, the small venules may show septal hemorrhage and a collection of radially arranged lymphocytes and histiocytes. Direct immunofluorescence studies at this early stage show deposition of immunoglobulins (Ig) IgM or IgG and complement products in the vessel walls. In time, mononuclear cells become more numerous and extend into lobular portion of the subcutis followed by septal fibrosis. Granulomas are not seen.

TREATMENT

In sarcoidosis, EN rarely needs any specific treatment. Almost all patients with EN recover spontaneously. Fever and troublesome arthralgias respond to bed rest and nonsteroidal anti-inflammatory agents.

Bed rest, elevation of the legs, elastic stockings, mild sedation, and analgesics may be necessary. Associated iridocyclitis should be treated appropriately with corticosteroids.[3-8]

CASE 1

A 25-year-old Irish woman, previously healthy, woke up in the morning with mild sore throat, fatigue, pain in both ankles, and red lesions on her legs. She had been unwell for the last two days, but denied fever, chills, nausea, and night sweats. She worked in a restaurant, does not take any recreational drugs or use oral contraceptives. She lived in London and has not traveled for 3 years.

Physical examination showed red tender bumps and blotches on both shins. The nodules were in the skin and were not movable. Ankles were mildly swollen and tender. Lungs, heart, and eyes were normal.

A chest X-ray film showed bilateral lower lobe infiltration (Figure 10-1). Her tuberculin skin test was negative. Thus, history, physical examination, chest X-ray finding, and negative tuberculin test excluded sarcoidosis, tuberculosis, brucellosis, coccidiodomycosis, histoplasmosis, and drug reaction. Complement fixation antibody titers were positive for psittacosis pneumonia.

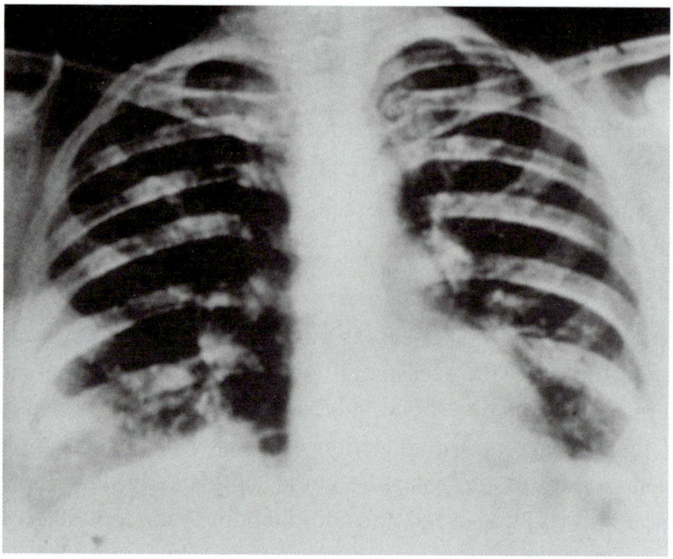

Figure 10-1 Chest X-ray with bilateral lower lobe infiltration representing psittacosis pneumonia.

CASE 2

This 28-year old woman from Barbados, who has lived in London for the last 10 years, woke up with red-eyes, photophobia, and nodules on the legs. She had no fever, malaise, cough, or joint pains. Her older sister had sarcoidosis.

Physical examination showed bilateral iritis and enlarged lachrymal glands (Figure 10-2).

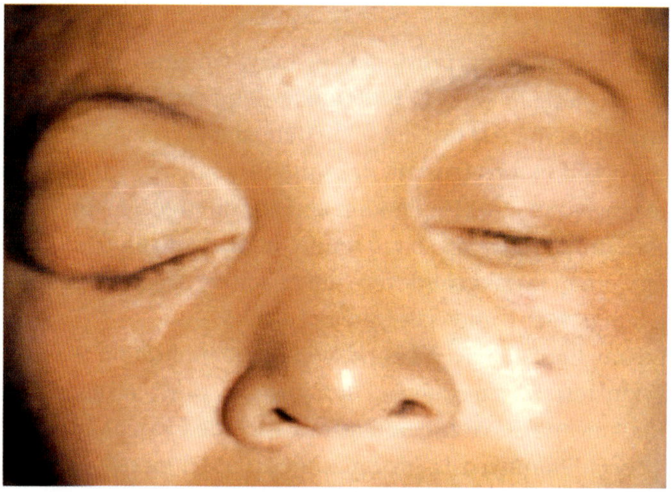

Figure 10-2 Enlarged lachrymal glands are not frequently noticed in patients with sarcoidosis.

Lungs and heart were normal. There were many dark lumps on her legs and lower parts of the thighs (Figure 10-3). Her tuberculin test was negative and serum angiotensin converting enzyme was elevated. A chest X-ray showed bilateral hilar adenopathy consistent with the diagnosis of sarcoidosis (Figure 10-4). The patient refused a mediastinal lymph node biopsy. This was the case of sarcoidosis; all the possible causes of EN were excluded (Figure 10-5). She was given corticosteroid eye drops for the eye inflammation. Bilateral hilar adenopathy subsided in about 9 months.

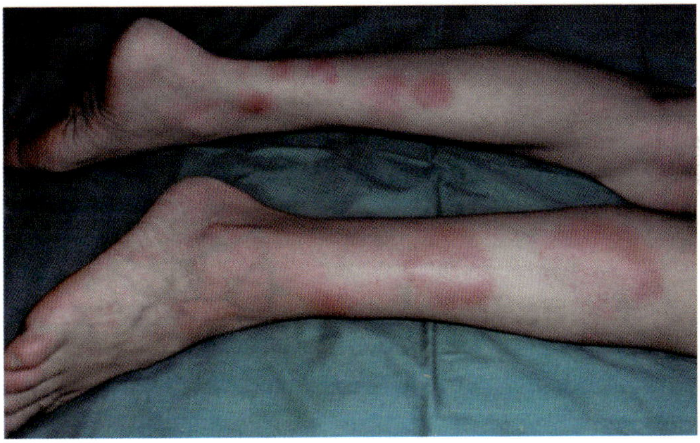

Figure 10-3 Erythema nodosum—the hallmark of acute sarcoidosis with large and rounded patches.

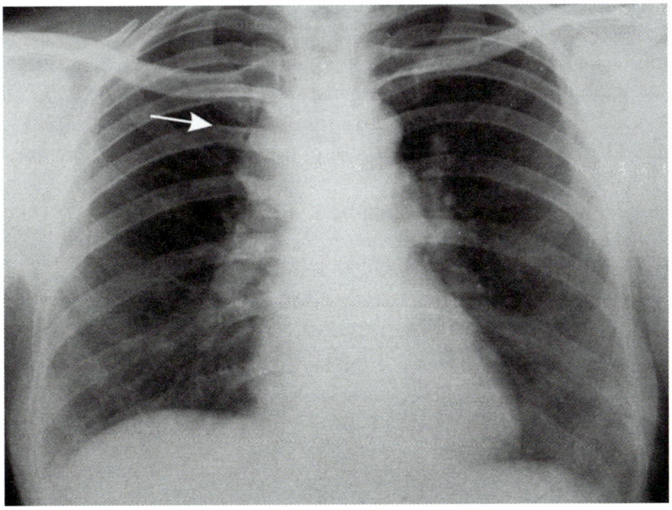

Figure 10-4 Bilateral hilar lymphadenopathy (BHL) with clear lung fields. BHL, the classic radiographic feature of sarcoidosis is present in nearly three quarters of patients; right paratracheal lymph nodes may be involved concomitantly (white arrow).

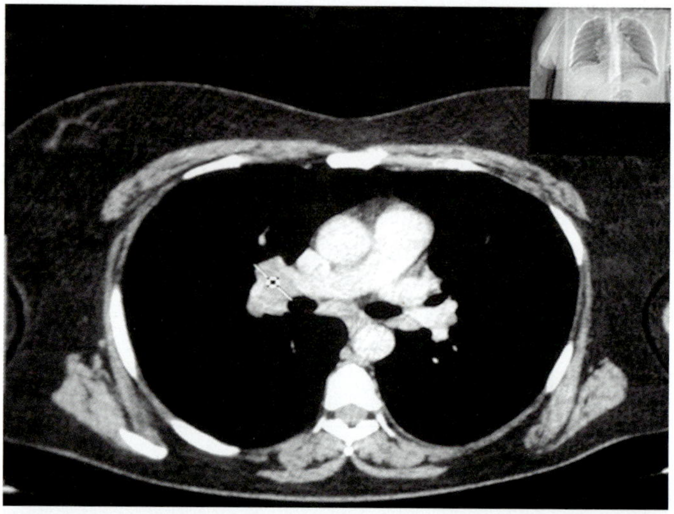

Figure 10-5 Characteristic features of sarcoidosis on computed tomography (CT) include mediastinal and/or hilar lymphadenopathy. However, despite the enhanced accuracy of CT, routine CT is not necessary or cost-effective in the management of sarcoidosis. Enlargement of left paratracheal, para-aortic, and subcarinal lymph node groups may be detected by CT scans, but are not usually evident on plain chest radiographs.

REFERENCES

1. Sharma O. Robert Willan Remembered. *J Am Acad Dermatol.* 1983;9:971-6.
2. Grunewald J, Eklund A. Sex-specific manifestations of Löfgren's syndrome. *Am J Resp Crit Care Med.* 2007;175:40-5.
3. Verma KK, Srivastava P, Minz A, Verma K. Role of azathioprine in preventing recurrences in a patient of recurrent erythema nodosum leprosum. *Lepr Rev.* 2006;77:225-9.
4. Saricaoglu H, Karadogan SK, Bayazit N, Yucel A, Dilek K, Tunali S. Clinical features of late-onset Behcet's disease: Report of 9 cases. *Int J Dermatol.* 2006;45:1284-7
5. Guerre-Schmidt AR, Pelletier F, Carbonnel F, Humbert P, Aubin F. Dermatosis-arthritis syndrome associated with Crohn's disease in a teenager. *Rev Med Interne.* 2006;27:847-7.
6. B'chir Hamzaoui S, Harmel A, Bouslama K, Abdallah M, Ennafaa M, M'rad S, et al; le groupe tunisien d'étude sur la maladie de Behçet. Behcet's disease in Tunisia. Clinical study of 519 cases. *Rev Med Interne.* 2006;27:742-50.
7. Jalava K, Hakkinen M, Valkonen M, Nakari UM, Palo T, Hallanvuo S, et al. An outbreak of gastrointestinal illness with erythema nodosum from grated carrots contaminated with Yersinia peudotuberculosis. *J Infect Dis.* 2006;104:1209-16.
8. Clayton TH, Walker BP, Stables GI. Treatment of chronic erythema nodosum with infliximab. *Clin Exp Dermatol.* 2006;31:823-4.

CHAPTER

11 Lacrimal Gland Enlargement

ANATOMY

Lacrimal glands are paired almond-shaped structures, one for each eye, located within the lacrimal fossa of the orbit formed by the frontal bone. The glands continually releases tears which cleanse, protect, lubricate, and moisten the eyes. The gland has 2 parts; the smaller palpebral portion and the larger orbital portion which contains fine interlobular ducts that form excretory ducts.

Tears secreted collect in the fornices pass over the eye surface to the lacrimal puncta, small holes found at the inner corner of the eyelids. The tears then pass on to the lacrimal sac, nasolacrimal duct, and out into the nose. Inflammation of the lacrimal glands is called dacryoadenitis.

HISTORY

Johann von Mikulicz was Professor of Surgery at Breslau. In 1892, he described a 42-year-old farmer with symmetrical enlargement of lacrimal and parotid glands, and dryness of the mouth.[1]

CLINICAL FEATURES OF LACRIMAL SARCOIDOSIS

In sarcoidosis, clinically symptomatic granulomatous infiltration of the lacrimal glands is not too frequent (Figure 11-1); however, gallium-67 scanning reveals significantly more patients with lacrimal involvement. Sulavik et al. analyzed the diagnostic sensitivity and specificity of gallium-67 uptake in the lacrimal, parotid, and hilar glands in sarcoidosis. The image produce by the gallium-67 uptake of the lacrimal and salivary glands resemble the face of a panda bear and is classified as panda pattern. The panda pattern was seen in 79% of the patients.[2] Dryness, swelling, and pain in the eyes are common symptoms. In asymptomatic patients, the decrease in lacrimal secretions can be diagnosed by Schrimer's test. Gallium-67 scanning for lacrimal glands is nonspecific because it may be positive in otherwise normal individuals.[3,4]

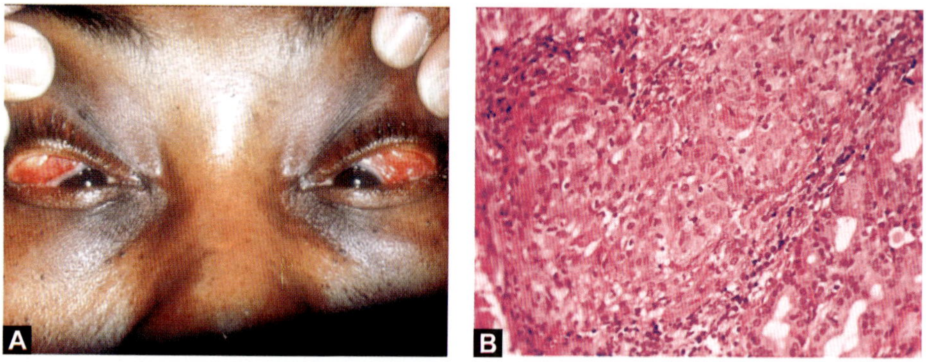

Figure 11-1 Lacrimal glands (bilateral) enlargement due to sarcoidosis. **A,** Lacrimal glands involvement. **B,** Biopsy revealed the diagnosis of sarcoidosis.

DIFFERENTIAL DIAGNOSIS

Tumors of the lacrimal glands are rare, but they can be life-threatening. There are three major categories of lacrimal gland tumors: primary epithelial, primary nonepithelial, and inflammatory. The common epithelial tumors are papilloma, squamous cell carcinoma, transitional cell-carcinoma, and plasmacytoma. The common primary nonepithelial tumors are fibrous histiocytoma, malignant lymphoma, and melanoma. The common inflammatory lesions are sarcoidosis, Wegener's granulomatosis, amyloidosis ulcerative colitis, and pyogenic granuloma.[5,6]

Immunoglobulin G4-related Systemic Disease and Eosinophilic Angiocentric Fibrosis

Immunoglobulin G4 (IgG-4) related systemic disease is a relatively new multisystem disease characterized by high serum IgG-4 levels and IgG-4 positive plasma cell infiltrate in involved tissues. The disease preferentially targets 2 organs: pancreas (autoimmune pancreatitis) and lacrimal and parotid glands. The cause is not known but this IgG-4 related systemic disease appears to be a phenotype of Mikulicz's syndrome. The disease responds to corticosteroids.[7-9]

Kuttner Tumor or Sclerosing Sialadenitis

In 1896, Kuttner reported 4 cases with the submandibular gland swellings. Histologically, they showed chronic inflammation and fibrosis. Sporadic cases of this entity have come to be known as Kuttner's tumor or chronic sclerosing sialadenitis of the submandibular gland. It is defined as a chronic inflammatory disease with recurrent swellings of the face and lacrimal glands. It is diagnosed chiefly histologically because there are no specific symptoms. The association has been underrecognized.[10]

TREATMENT AND PROGNOSIS

The course of lacrimal gland sarcoidosis is similar to that of intrathoracic sarcoidosis. Response to corticosteroids is good.

REFERENCES

1. Mikulicz J. Beitrage Zur Chirurgie: Festschrift Theodore Billroth. Sttutgart: 1892. p. 610.
2. Sulavik S, Spencer RB, Weed DA, Shapiro HR, Shiue ST, Castriotta RJ. Recognition of distinctive patterns of gallium-67 distribution in sarcoidosis. *J Nucl Med.* 1990;31:1909-14.
3. Ross AH, Herbert HM, Kabala J, Malhotra R. Lacrimal uptake of gallium (67Ga) citrate in patients without ocular pathology. *Orbit.* 2009;28:120-3.
4. Heindl LM, Jünemann AG, Kruse FE, Holbach LM. Tumors of the lacrimal drainage system. *Orbit.* 2010;29:298-306.
5. Mochizuki K, Sawada A, Katsumura N. Case of lacrimal gland inflammation associated with ulcerative colitis. *Int Ophthalmol.* 2010;30:109-11.
6. Lim EJ, Bhathal PS, Tagkalidis PP, Speer AG. Catching a chameleon: IgG4-related systemic disease. *Med J Aust.* 2010;193:418-20.
7. Takahashi H, Yamamoto M, Suzuki C, Naishiro Y, Shinomura Y, Imai K. The birthday of a new syndrome: IgG-4 related diseases constitute a clinical entity. *Autoimmun Rev.* 2010;9:591-4.
8. Ho HW, Lin Z, T Lim KH, Choo CT. Bilateral Kuttner tumours of the lacrimal glands. *Orbit.* 2011;30:96-7.
9. Shigemitsu H, Koss MN. IgG4-related interstitial lung disease: a new and evolving concept. *Curr Opin Pulm Med.* 2009;15:513-6.
10. Sánchez-Acosta A, Moreno-Arredondo D, Rubio-Solornio RI, Rodríguez-Martínez HA, Rodríguez-Reyes AA. Angio-lymphoid hyperplasia with eosinophilia of the lacrimal gland: a case report. *Orbit.* 2008;27:195-8.

CHAPTER

12 Bilateral Hilar Adenopathy

INCIDENCE

Bilateral hilar adenopathy (BHL) is the earliest chest roentgenographic abnormality, occurring in more than 50% of all patients with sarcoidosis. ymph node enlargement primarily involves the bronchopulmonary, tracheabronchial, and paratracheal nodes. There is a translucent space between the enlarged nodes and the cardiovascular margin. Because the hilum is better visible on the right, the "space" is clearer on the right side. Hilar adenopathy may be associated with either right paratracheal (25%) or bilateral paratracheal lymph node enlargement (Figures 12-1 to 12-5). The "one-two-three" sign of bilateral and right paratracheal adenopathy is considered classic for the disease. Gallium uptake by this group of lymph nodes is called lambda sign.

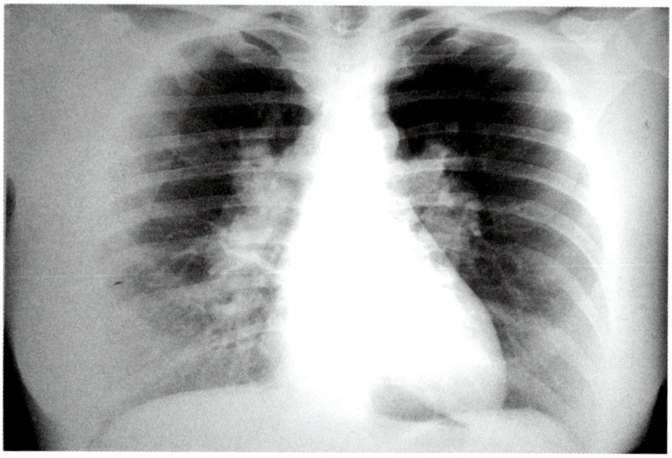

Figure 12-1 These enlarged lymph nodes are classically located in both hila, in the pre- and right-paratracheal mediastinum, in the aortopulmonary window, in the subcarinal area and, less frequently, in the anterior and posterior mediastinum. However, only the right paratracheal and hilar lymph nodes and those located in the aortic pulmonary window can easily identified on a posteroanterior chest radiograph.

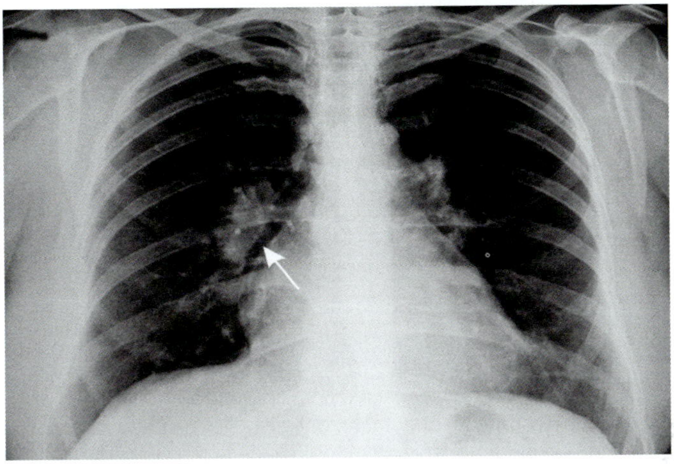

Figure 12-2 There is a translucent space between the enlarged nodes and the cardiovascular margin, because the hilum is better visible on the right the "space" is clearer on the right side.

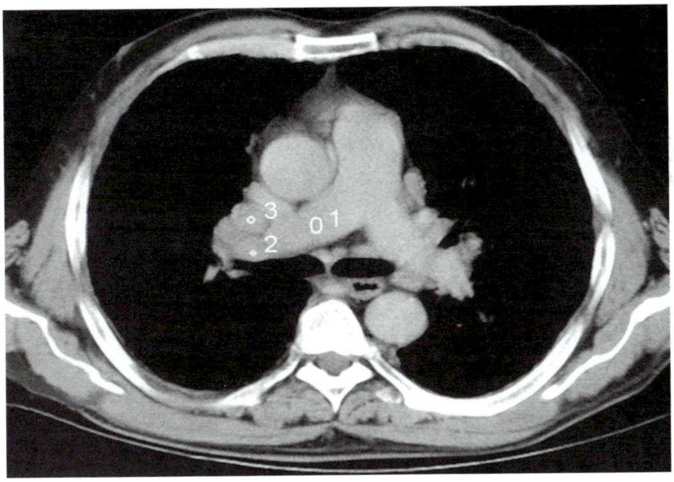

Figure 12-3 Axial computed tomography image in a patient with sarcoidosis. Enlarged lymph nodes can be seen in the mediastinum and in both hila.

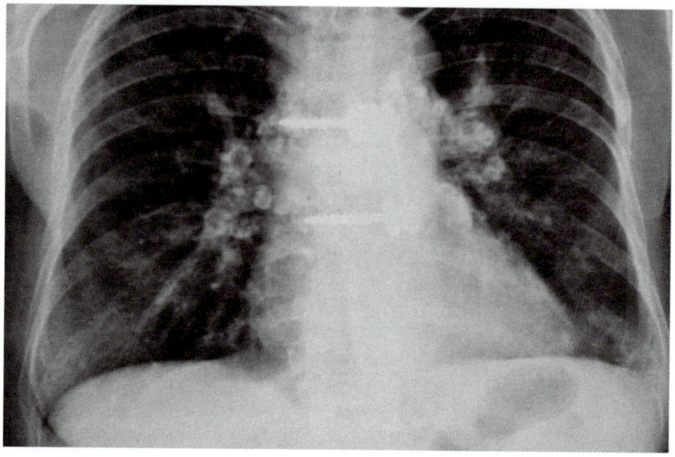

Figure 12-4 Calcification can occur in affected nodes, especially in patients with longstanding sarcoidosis, and can be amorphous, punctuate, or eggshell. The chest radiograph belongs to a patient with the diagnosis of pulmonary sarcoidosis made in the year 2000. The vertebral bone fracture which occurred in 2002 was due to sarcoidosis of the vertebral bones (histological finding at the operation). Visible metal shadow belongs to the metal graft (vertebral implant) used to stabilize the vertebral bones.

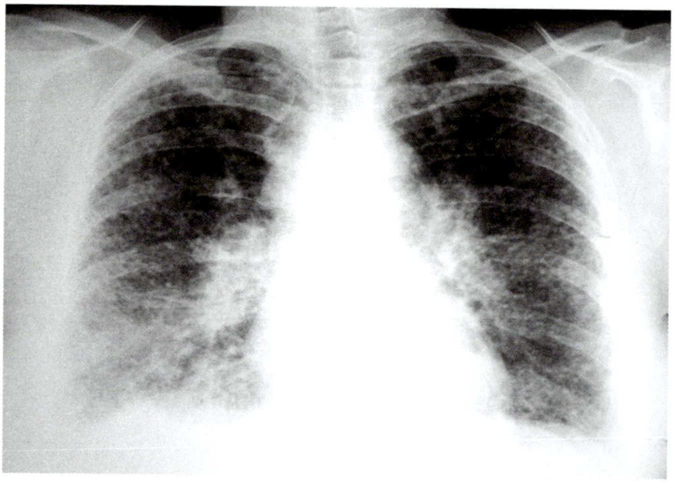

Figure 12-5 Approximately 10–15% of the patients with stage I disease may remain stationary or advance only slowly to stage II. The chest X-ray representing stage II with parenchymal lesions but the bilateral hilar adenopathy is still clearly visible.

CLINICAL FEATURES

Bilateral hilar adenopathy is the hallmark of acute, early reversible sarcoidosis, particularly if associated with erythema nodosum. The differential diagnosis of BHL (stage I) sarcoidosis includes lymphoma, primary tuberculosis, coccidioidomycosis,

Table 12-1 Causes of Bilateral Hilar Adenopathy/Fullness

Common	*Uncommon*	*Rare*
Sarcoidosis	Tuberculosis	Brucellosis
Lymphoma	Histoplasmosis	Infectious mononucleosis
Pneumoconiosis	Coccidioidomycosis	Amyloidosis
Bronchogenic carcinoma	Dilantin	Leukemia
Lymph node metastases	Methotrexate	
Pulmonary hypertension	Schistosomiasis	

histoplasmosis, brucellosis, metastatic lymph node involvement due to lung, testicular, renal, breast, and colon carcinomas (Table 12-1). The symmetrical enlargement of hilar lymph nodes in an asymptomatic person or one with erythema nodosum or iridocyclitis is rarely due to anything but sarcoidosis. The Kveim-Siltzbach test is positive in about 65% of the cases.

Bilateral paratracheal adenopathy as the sole abnormality, unilateral adenopathy, and mediastinal adenopathy without hilar adenopathy are rarely seen in sarcoidosis.

DIFFERENTIAL DIAGNOSIS

After analyzing 100 patients, Winterbauer et al.[1] found that hilar adenopathy in an asymptomatic patient with negative physical examination or in association with erythema nodosum or uveitis constitutes a strong evidence of sarcoidosis. However, bilateral hilar adenopathy in association with anemia, pleural effusion, anterior mediastinal mass, peripheral adenopathy, or hepatomegaly may represent either a neoplasm or lymphoma and need tissue diagnosis. Mediastinal adenopathy in Hodgkin's disease tends to be localized in the anterior and superior mediastinum with a lesser tendency to resemble the "scalloped" or "potato" bronchopulmonary nodes due to sarcoidosis. Tuberculosis is in the differential diagnosis (Figures 12-6 and 12-7); however, it should be realized that active

Table 12-2 Causes of Unilateral Hilar Adenopathy/Fullness

Common	*Uncommon*
Primary tuberculosis	Sarcoidosis
Primary coccidioidomycosis	Amyloidosis
Lymphoma	Aneurysm of a pulmonary artery
Histoplasmosis	Pulmonary embolism
Pulmonary artery stenosis	Poststenotic pulmonary art dilatation
Apical segment (lower lobe) lesions	Schistosomiasis

tuberculosis is diagnosed in only 1–2% of the patients with hilar adenopathy. In tuberculosis, coccidioidomycosis, and lung neoplasm, the adenopathy is usually unilateral (Table 12-2).

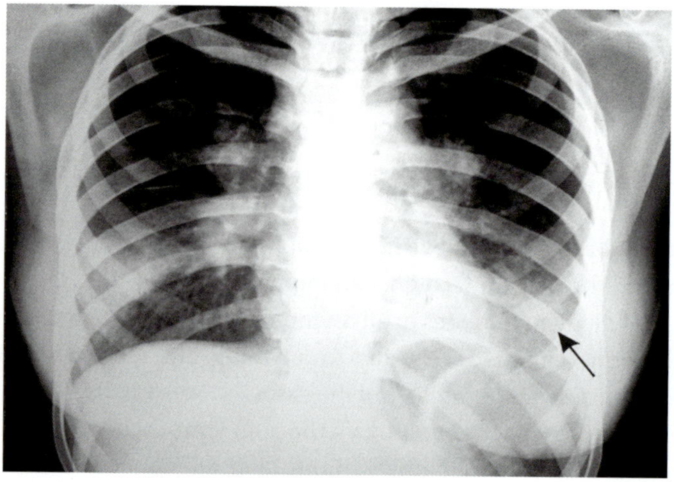

Figure 12-6 The chest X-ray representing bilateral hilar adenopathy. Minimal pleural effusion at the left side (arrow). However, this was not sarcoidosis; the most troublesome differential diagnosis, especially in the countries with high incidence of tuberculosis. The chest X-ray from a patient with primary tuberculosis. She was 20 years old student from Kenya where the incidence of tuberculosis exceeds 300/100,000. No Bacillus Calmette-Guérin vaccination. The diagnosis of tuberculosis was obtained by smear positive and Lowenstein positive sputum culture.

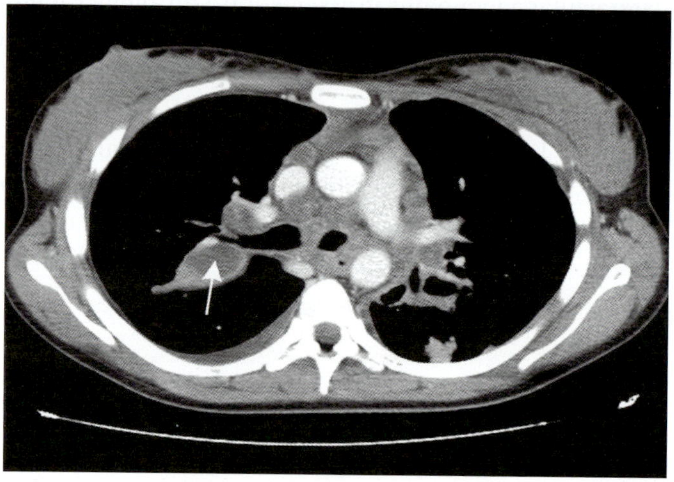

Figure 12-7 Computed tomography scan of the same patient. The structure of the lymph nodes almost suggesting the diagnosis (zones of necrosis arrow).

COURSE

In 60–80% of the patients with only bilateral hilar adenopathy, complete or substantial clearing occurs with 2 years. Once the lymph nodes subside spontaneously, they rarely, if ever, enlarge again. About 10% of the patients follow a persistent course. This small group has chronic skin lesions and bone cysts. The remaining 10–15% of the patients with stage I disease may remain stationary or advance only slowly to stage II. The combination of erythema nodosum and bilateral hilar adenopathy called Lofgren's syndrome predicts a favorable outcome of sarcoidosis. The hilar enlargement is characteristically symmetrical, although a larger number of lymph nodes on the right side may produce an impression of pronounced right-sided enlargement. The improved prognosis in patients with erythema nodosum is limited to the white sarcoidosis population.[2]

TREATMENT

The patients with asymptomatic bilateral hilar adenopathy with or without erythema nodosum require no treatment.

Computed tomography (CT) examination is usually necessary to show the involvement of the other node groups. Although contrast-enhanced CT can better distinguish enlarged lymph nodes from the vascular structures in the mediastinum, and especially in the hila, injection of contrast is not always necessary to make the diagnosis. Mediastinal adenopathy without hilar involvement or with unilateral hilar involvement is rare but can be seen especially in older patients.[3]

REFERENCES

1. Winterbauer RH, Belic M, Moores KD. Clinical interpretation of bilateral hilar adenopathy. *Ann Intern Med.* 1973;78:65-71.
2. Mihailovic-Vucinic V, Sharma OP. Atlas of Sarcoidosis: pathogenesis, diagnosis and clinical features. London: Springer; 2005.
3. Rockoff SD, Rohatgi PK. Unusual manifestations of thoracic sarcoidosis. *AJR Am J Roentgenol.* 1985;144:513-28.

CHAPTER

13 Darier-Roussy Syndrome (Subcutaneous Sarcoidosis)

DEFINITION

Darier-Roussy syndrome or Darier-Roussy disease, an uncommon subcutaneous manifestation of sarcoidosis was first described by Darier and Roussy in 1904.[1] The lesion is characterized by numerous 0.5–0.3 cm deep-seated nodules on the trunk and extremities.

HISTORY

Ferdinand-Jean Darier was born in Budapest, Hungary to French parents. He was the contemporary of the most outstanding figures of the medical fraternity at the beginning of the 20th century. Darier was one of the "big five" scientists of his time, along with Ernest Henri Besnier (1831–1909), Louis-Anne-Jean Brocq (1856–1928), Raymond Sabouraud (1864–1938), and Jean Alfred Fournier (1832–1915), working in the famous Paris School of Dermatology.

During his work, Darier discovered several dermatological diseases describing them as follicular psorodermose, follicular keratosis, acanthosis nigricans, dermatofibrosarcoma, and erythema annularis. Nowadays, well-known typical skin lesion of chronic sarcoidosis—subcutaneous sarcoidosis or Darier-Roussy sarcoid, was also described by Ferdinand-Jean Darier and his French colleague Gustave Roussy.

Gustave Roussy studied medicine at the University of Geneva, Lausanne and then moved to Paris to continue his studies at the Faculté de Medicine. Despite the war time (World War I), Roussy was a very productive scientist. He was well known for his fundamental research on neurology, especially the functions of the autonomic nervous system, as well as the textbook about war psychosis.

Gustav Roussy worked as a professor of pathology at the faculty of medicine in Paris, later on as a director of the Cancer Institute. In 1933, Roussy worked as a dean of the Medical Faculty, University of Paris, and in 1937, became its rector. He was also an honorary member and an honorary doctor in several European universities of Geneva, Lausanne, Athens, and Budapest.

CLINICAL FEATURES

Subcutaneous sarcoidosis or Darier-Roussy sarcoid is represented by numerous deep-seated nodules on the trunk and extremities.[1-4] Rarely, subcutaneous sarcoidosis occurs in patients without evidence of systemic disease. Darier-Roussy lesions can be localized as single solitary large lesion of 4–6 inch in diameter, but commonly the nodules are many, of varying sizes from 0.5–2 cm in diameter (Figure 13-1). Commonly found over the trunk and extremities, the lesions are more prominent near the bony prominences. Face can also be involved. The nodules are painless, firm, and freely movable without overlying epidermal involvement. When superficial, they may acquire a bluish hue; ulceration is rare.

In their large retrospective case study, examining the clinical and pathologic characteristics of patients with subcutaneous sarcoidosis, Ahmed and Harshad found 33 cases described in the literature and added 21 new cases from their own institutional database.[5] The authors noted a peak incidence of subcutaneous sarcoidosis in the 4th decade of life in the analyzed study population. In addition,

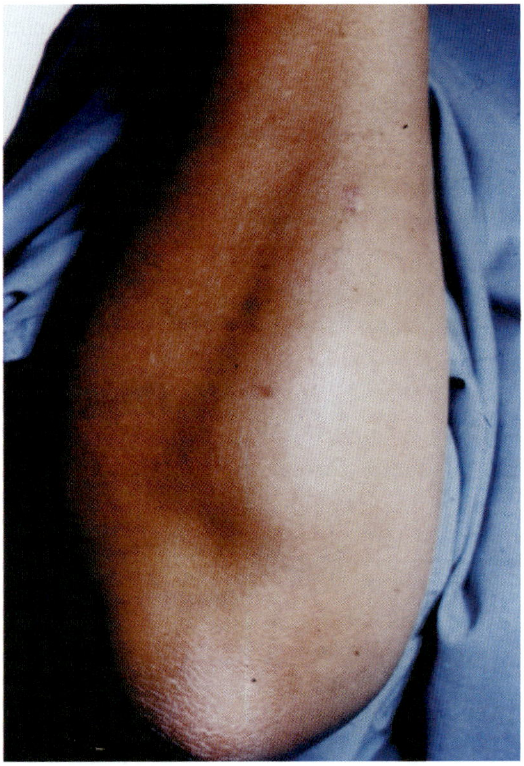

Figure 13-1 Darier-Roussy lesion as a single solitary large lesion of 2–3 inch in diameter. This patient is treated with corticosteroids and methotrexate due to chronic persistent pulmonary sarcoidosis.

there was a slightly higher incidence in female patients as compared to male patients from this study.[5] The authors also found an association between subcutaneous sarcoidosis and autoimmune diseases. The associations have been already described in literature including vitiligo, pernicious anemia, and autoimmune thyroiditis.[6]

Another smaller retrospective review of 10 patients with subcutaneous sarcoidosis done by Marcoval et al., however, showed the peak incidence in the 5th and 6th decades of life.[7]

DIAGNOSIS

The diagnosis of subcutaneous sarcoidosis is made in the presence of subcutaneous epithelioid granulomas with multinucleated giant cells and extracutaneous systemic disease involvement, especially bilateral hilar adenopathy. In some patients, the occurrence of subcutaneous sarcoidosis has also been described in the absence of systemic disease.

DIFFERENTIAL DIAGNOSIS

Lesions similar to Darier-Roussy sarcoidosis can be seen in tuberculosis and sometimes syphilis. The parasitic lesions of the "Calabar swellings" of filaria *Loa-loa* infestations are indistinguishable from subcutaneous sarcoid lesions. Named after Calabar, a Nigerian seaport, these lesions are localized swollen lumps of subcutaneous tissue caused by a parasitic filarial worm *Loa-loa* endemic to Central and West Africa. The swollen areas migrate with the worm through the body at a speed of about 1 cm/minute and may become as large as a small egg. *Onchocerca volvulus* is a nematode that causes skin nodules and long-term corneal inflammation, or keratitis, mostly in Africa.

Skin and subcutaneous metastatic lesions from carcinomas, particularly breast and lymphoma can look like subcutaneous sarcoidosis, leading to misdiagnosis.

Occasionally, a lipoma, as a growth of fat cells just below the skin surface can resemble Darier-Roussy nodule. However, the predilection places of lipomas are the torso, neck, upper thighs, upper arms, and armpits; while Darier-Roussy subcutaneous nodules are usually found on the trunk and extremities.

Vasculitis, Madelung's disease, and related lipomatous disorders can also produce subcutaneous nodules.

PATHOLOGY

The subcutaneous sarcoidosis lesions show typical epithelioid noncaseating granulomas in the subcutaneous tissue. The nodules occur in the deep dermis and in the fat tissue. Appropriate tests, special stains, and cultures must be obtained to exclude tuberculosis, fungal, and parasitic organisms. Calcification is rare.

TREATMENT

Oral corticosteroids are the mainstay of treatment. When we used prednisone 20 mg/day; response was noted within 4–8 weeks. Methotrexate or hydroxychloroquine are used if there are too many side effects of corticosteroid therapy. Many other treatment options have also been reported.[5-10]

REFERENCES

1. James WD, Berger TG. Andrews' diseases of the skin: clinical dermatology. Philadelphia: Saunders Elsevier; 2006.
2. Vainsencher D, Winkelmann RK. Subcutaneous sarcoidosis. *Arch Dermatol.* 1984;120:1028-31.
3. Shapiro PE. Noninfectious granulomas. In: Elder D, Elenitsas R, Johnson BL, Murphy GF, Xu X, editors. Lever's Histopathology of the Skin. 8th ed. Philadelphia: Lippincott-Raven; 1997. p. 323.
4. Howard A, White CR. Non-infectious granulomas. In: Bolognia JL, Joizzo JL, Schaffer JV, editors. Dermatology. New York: Mosby; 2003. p. 1455.
5. Ahmed I, Harshad SR. Subcutaneous sarcoidosis: is it a specific subset of cutaneous sarcoidosis frequently associated with systemic disease? *J Am Acad Dermatol.* 2006;54:55-60.
6. Barnadas MA, Rodríguez-Arias JM, Alomar A. Subcutaneous sarcoidosis associated with vitiligo, pernicious anemia and autoimmune thyroiditis. *Clin Exp Dermatol.* 2000;25:55-6.
7. Marcoval J, Maña J, Moreno A, Peyri J. Subcutaneous sarcoidosis--clinicopathological study of 10 cases. *Br J Dermatol.* 2005;153:790-4.
8. Voelter-Mahlknecht S, Benez A, Metzger S, Fierlbeck G. Treatment of subcutaneous sarcoidosis with allopurinol. *Arch Dermatol.* 1999;135:1560-1.
9. Bachelez H, Senet P, Cadranel J, Kaoukhov A, Dubertret L. The use of tetracyclines for the treatment of sarcoidosis. *Arch Dermatol.* 2001;137:69-73.
10. Fichtel JC, Duckworth AK, Soares T, Lesher JL Jr. Subcutaneous sarcoidosis presenting after treatment of Cushing's disease. *J Am Acad Dermatol.* 2006;54:360-1.

CHAPTER

14 Lupus Pernio

DEFINITION

Lupus pernio is the most typical and easily recognizable skin lesions of sarcoidosis. It is a bluish, violaceous red induration that affects the nose and the vicinal areas.

Ernest Besnier, in 1889, gave the lesion its unusual name and distinguished it from the lesion of tuberculosis called lupus vulgaris.[1]

HISTORY

On February 14, 1889, Ernest Besnier, Chief of Medicine and one of the grand men of French Dermatology presented a case entitled, *"Lupus Pernio of the Face- symmetrical scrofulo-tuberculosis of the upper extremities"*. The lecture began, "Here is man, aged 34 years, who exhibits lesions of the same type in both face and upper extremities, although with differing appearances in each, which are not well understood or described. First the face represents lupus erythematosus, which I propose to name lupus pernio or lupus asphyxiation, similar to Hutchinson's chilblains, but not identical." In describing lupus pernio, Besnier clearly differentiated the lesion from other dermatological conditions, including tuberculosis.[1,2]

INCIDENCE

In the United States, the lesion is more frequent in African-American women than in Caucasian patients. In the United Kingdom, lupus pernio is more common in women of West Indian origin. The lesion is associated with chronic multisystem disease in many systems, particularly in the bones.[3]

CLINICAL FEATURES AND COURSE

Lupus pernio is a chronic lesion that has a predilection for nose, cheeks, and ears. Its appearance ranges from a few small button-like nodules under the tip of the nose to exuberant plaques covering the nose and spreading across the cheeks (Figure 14-1). Occasionally, there are similar nodules on the eyelids and ears and associated plaques on the arms, buttocks, and thighs. Lupus pernio is an indicator of chronic fibrotic sarcoidosis in all affected systems. It develops insidiously and progresses indolently over many years. It can be complicated by nasal septal perforation, which may be aggravated disastrously by the well-meaning intervention of nasal and plastic surgeons. Bone cysts are occasionally present in the small bones of the hands (Figure 14-2) and feet.

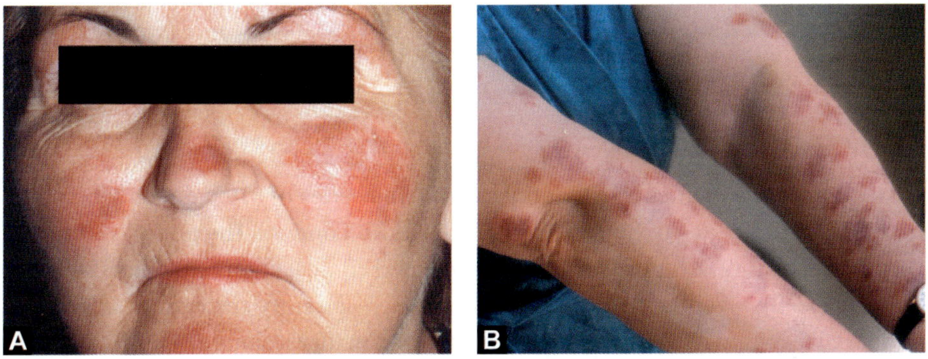

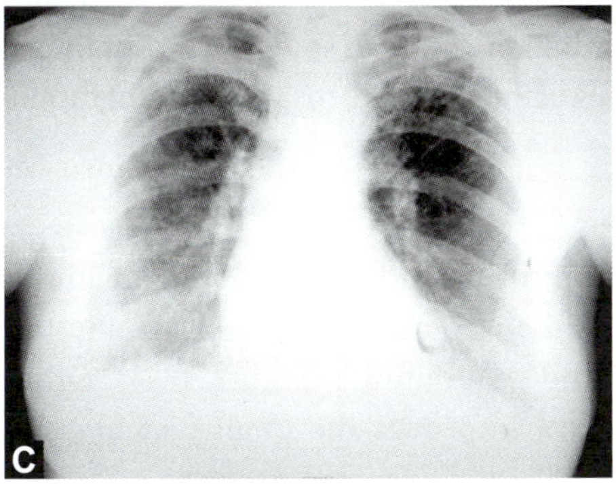

Figure 14-1 A, A 63-year-old lady presented to the clinic with cutaneous lesions resembling lupus pernio on her face. **B,** She also had associated plaques on the arms, buttocks, and thighs. **C,** Chest X-ray of the same patient presenting stage III of lung sarcoidosis (fibrotic lesions, with hilar retraction).

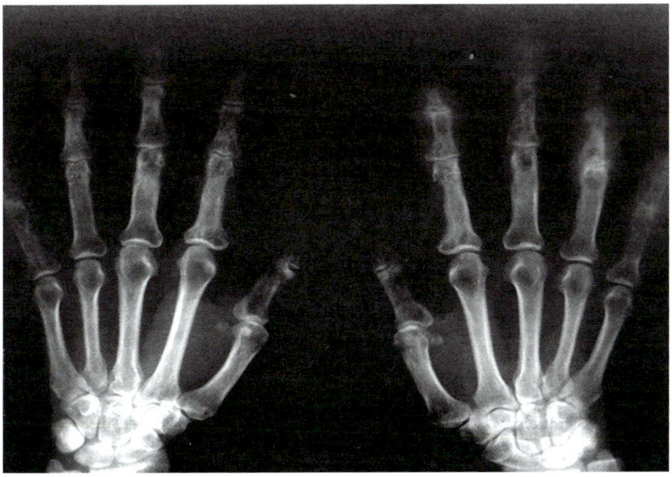

Figure 14-2 X-ray of hand showing multiple bone cysts in the above patient with lupus pernio.

Occasionally, lupus pernio may resemble cutaneous lesions of leprosy, necrotizing vasculitis, leprosy, coccidioidomycosis, blastomycosis, systemic lupus erythematosus, lymphoma, and rhinophyma. Lupus pernio rarely ulcerate and rarely turn into fungating masses.

HISTOLOGY

Biopsies of the skin, nose, and nasal mucosa show typical noncaseating granulomas (Figure 14-3).

COURSE AND PROGNOSIS

James reported 35 patients with lupus pernio in a series of 818 patients seen at the Sarcoidosis Clinic at the Royal Northern Hospital, London. The analysis provided the natural history of lupus pernio and associated clinical and radiological features. Lungs were involved in 74% of patients, upper respiratory tract in 54%, reticulo-endothelial system in 54%, bone cysts in 43%, and ocular lesions in 37%.[4]

Lupus pernio is a convenient experimental model to assess clinical course and response of therapy in sarcoidosis. In a single patient, one can study the morphologic appearance of the lesion, histological features of the nasal mucosa, and radiographic changes of the nasal bone erosion.[5]

TREATMENT

The treatment of lupus pernio needs to be prolonged, aggressive, and under continuous supervision. The drugs commonly used are corticosteroids, methotrexate, hydroxychloroquine, infliximab, and thalidomide (Figure 14-4). Other drugs are less helpful. Cosmetic camouflage improves the quality of life and social comfort.[6]

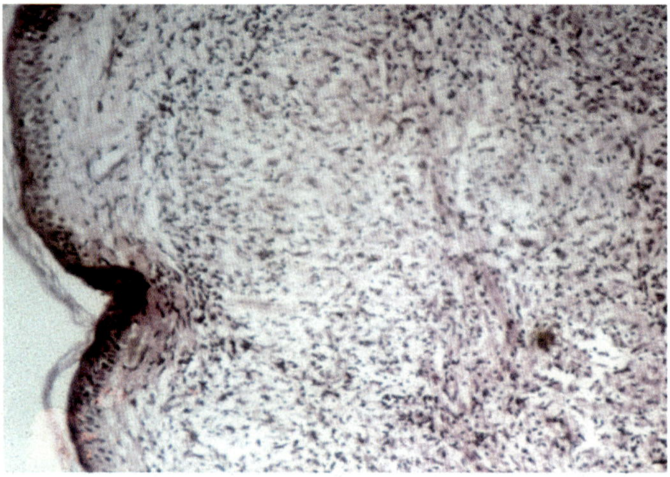

Figure 14-3 Skin biopsy revealed noncaseating sarcoid granulomas in the above patient.

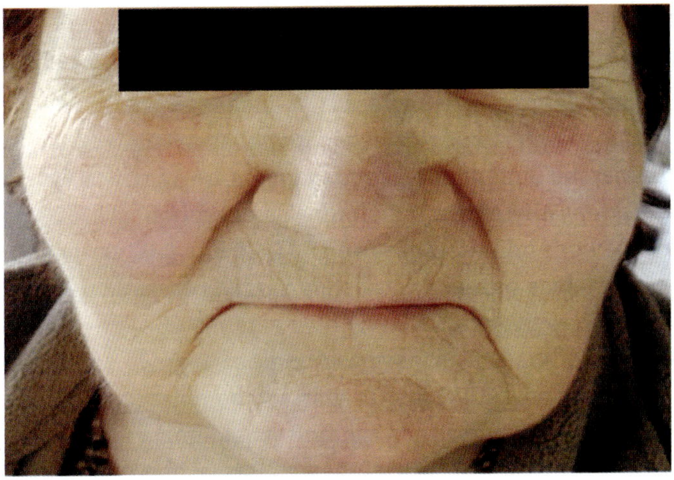

Figure 14-4 The above patient 12 years later. After years of therapy: the skin lesions remitted. She was treated with steroid therapy and methotrexate.

CASE STUDY

Mrs Am Verrant had chronic sarcoidosis: lupus pernio, bone involvement, blindness due to chronic uveitis, facial palsy, and pulmonary fibrosis (Figure 14-5). She has had sarcoidosis for about 70 years. She died at the age of 92 years and did not die of sarcoidosis but with it. Sarcoidosis patients can live a full life with small dose of prednisone. Patients need not be frightened unnecessarily for the long-lasting treatment.

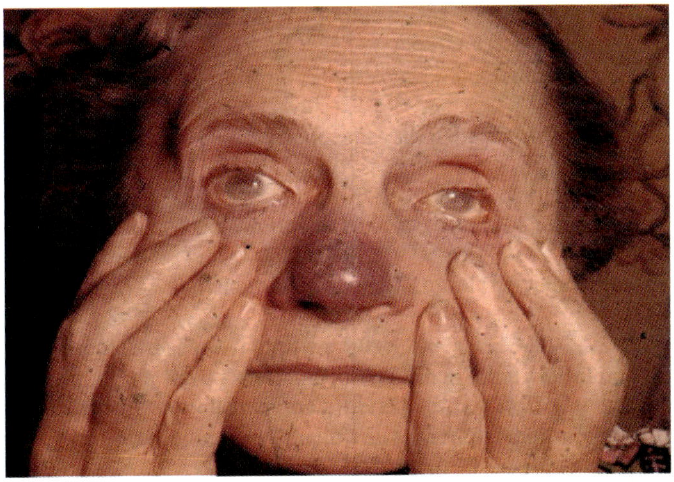

Figure 14-5 The history of this patient illustrates excellently what is already known about lupus pernio and what remains to be said.

REFERENCES

1. Turiaf J. Ernest Besnier (1831-1909) Et Lucien-Marie Pautrier (1876-1959). In: Levinský L, Macholda F, editors. Fifth International Conference on Sarcoidosis. Prague: University of Karlova; 1971. p. 57–62.
2. Hutchinson J. Case of Livid papillary psoriasis. Illustrations of Clinical Surgery. London: J & A Churchill Ltd.; 1877. p. 42.
3. James DG. Sarcoidosis and Other Granulomatous Disorders. Major Problems in Internal Medicine. Philadelphia; W.B. Saunders Co.; 1985. p. 24.
4. James D. Lupus pernio is a valuable experimental model. Sarcoidosis: Ninth International Conference on Sarcoidosis and Other Granulomatous Disorders. Paris: Pergamon Press; 1981. p. 465-9.
5. James DG. Lupus Pernio. Lupus. 1992;1:129-31.
6. Baughman RP, Lower EE. Evidence-based therapy for cutaneous sarcoidosis. *Clin Dermatol.* 2007;25:334-40.

CHAPTER

15 Parotid Gland Syndromes

ANATOMY

The parotid gland is the largest of the 3 major salivary glands. Enclosed within a capsule, it lies in an irregular bed located on the lateral aspect of the face. The 7th cranial (facial) nerve divides the gland into a large supraneural portion and a small infraneural component. One or both parotid glands may become enlarged in many infectious, inflammatory, and neoplastic diseases.

HISTORY

Christian Frederick Heerford (1871–1953) was a Danish ophthalmologist who first pointed out the association between uveitis and enlarged parotid glands, and called it "febris uveoparotidea chronica". He believed that mumps was the cause of the association. Heerfordt was born at Terndtrup, Denmark on December 26, 1871, son of a local doctor; he attended the Copenhagen University. As a keen European, he argued that Scandinavia and Europe should form a single community.[1]

In 1937, Jam Costa Waldenstrom (1906–1996) first recognized parotid enlargement as one of the manifestations of sarcoidosis. Born in Stockholm, he obtained his MD degree at the University of Uppsala. He was a professor of theoretical medicine at the University of Uppsala in 1941, professor of practical medicine at the University of Lund in 1944, and the head of the Department of Medicine at Malmö General Hospital until his retirement in 1972. In 1944, he described the disease that is now called Waldenstrom's macroglobulinema. His other contributions included studies on porphyrias, benign hypergammaglobulinemic purpura, chronic active hepatitis, pulmonary hemosiderosis, Bruton's hypogammaglobulinemia, paraneoplastic phenomena, carcinoid syndrome, and classification of gammopathies. He was a member of the National Academy of Science in the United States, the French Academy of Sciences, and was an honorary member of the Royal Society of Medicine, London.

Henrik Sjogren (1899–1986) was a Swedish ophthalmologist. With his wife, also an ophthalmologist, he collected a series of patients with dry eyes and mouth which he described in a 1933 thesis. There were 19 patients, all female, aged between 29 and 72, who had dry eyes and mouth and 13 of whom had a chronic arthritis. Now we classify Sjogren's syndrome as primary with no other clearly identifiable associated disease and secondary, where another disease, usually rheumatoid arthritis is present. Parotid involvement may occur in 25–55% of cases with Sjogren's syndrome. Unlike sarcoidosis, the risk of developing non-Hodgkin lymphoma is very high.

In 1892, Jan Mikulicz-Radecki recorded the first case of relapsing nonsuppurative relapsing parotid swellings. During the years that followed, a variety of unrelated conditions causing enlargement of the parotid glands were grouped together under the name Mikulicz' syndrome, with no regard to the histopathologic picture. Morgan and Castleman defined the changes consisting of unique diffuse infiltration with lymphocytes, alteration of the ducts, and hyalinization and fibrosis. Many of these cases were most likely due to sarcoidosis, lymphoma, and tuberculosis.[2,3]

CLINICAL FEATURES

In 1894, William Osler described an 11-year old African-American girl with enlarged parotid and lacrimal glands. The diagnosis of sarcoidosis was not entertained because the disease was not recognized at that time.[4] In retrospect, however, it appears that sarcoidosis was the most likely diagnosis. The parotid enlargement is now recognized as an important feature of sarcoidosis (Figure 15-1). Clinical manifestation of salivary gland enlargement occurs in less than <10% of the cases of sarcoidosis; however, histological evidence of noncaseating granulomas in more than one-third of the patients with sarcoidosis.[5] In a series of 537 patients seen at the Royal Northern Hospital, London, 33 (6%) had parotid gland enlargement. It was bilateral in 24 (73%), right sided in 6, and left sided in 3 patients. It occurred more commonly in women between 20- and 40-year age group. There was evidence of

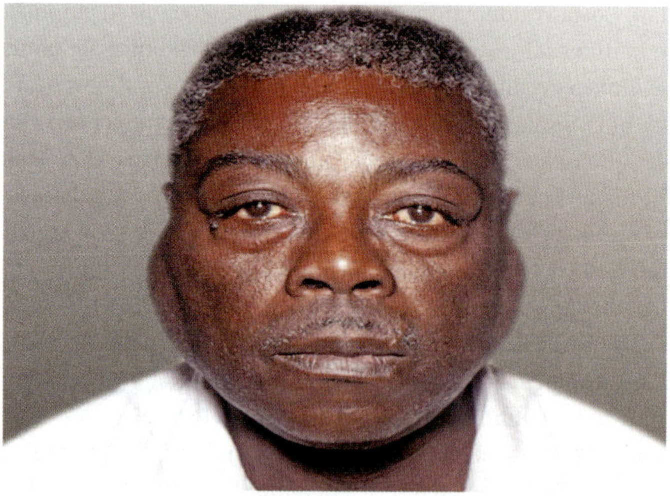

Figure 15-1 Sarcoid parotitis may be asymptomatic but is otherwise characterized by symptomatic enlargement of the parotid gland that is usually bilateral and results in the symptom of mouth dryness.

Table 15-1	Common Causes of Parotid Gland Enlargement
Infections	Tuberculosis, toxoplasmosis, histoplasmosis, cat scratch disease, and actinomycosis
Non-inflammatory	Sialosis/sialadenitis
Neoplasms	Lymphoma and adenoma
Drugs	Iodides
Miscellaneous	Melkersson-Rosenthal syndrome and liver failure

multisystem involvement, particularly the lungs, lymph nodes, eyes, skin lesions, and lacrimal glands.[2]

Heerfordt syndrome is chronic parotid gland enlargement and uveitis; occasionally facial nerve palsy is also a feature. In James' series, Heerfordt syndrome occurred in 19 patients; in 5, facial nerve palsy was also present. The fact that facial nerve palsy is so infrequent argues that it is not due to pressure from the enlarged parotid gland.[1]

DIFFERENTIAL DIAGNOSIS

The diagnosis of sarcoidosis is usually clear-cut in view of the typical bilateral parotid enlargement in patient with multisystem histologically confirmed sarcoidosis. A biopsy of salivary gland is rarely needed. Occasionally, other causes of parotid enlargement need to be considered (Table 15-1).[5]

COURSE AND PROGNOSIS

The course of parotid gland sarcoidosis in Heerfordt's syndrome is similar to that of intrathoracic sarcoidosis. No therapy is needed for asymptomatic parotitis. In 16 of 19 of James' patients, there was spontaneous resolution within 6 months, only 3 needed corticosteroids.[1,6] Surgery is rarely required.

REFERENCES

1. Waldenström JC. Some observations on uveoparotitis and allied conditions with special reference to the symptoms from the nervous system. *J Intern Med.* 1937:91;53-68.
2. James DG, Williams WJ. Sarcoidosis and other granulomatous disorders. Major Problems in Internal Medicine. Philadelphia: Saunders; 1985. Vol. 24.
3. Shearn MA. The Sjogren-Mikulicz syndrome—its relationship to connective tissue disorders. *Calif Med.* 1961;95:159-62.
4. Morgan WS, Castleman B. A clinicopathologic study of "Mikulicz's Disease". *Am J Pathol.* 1953;29:471-503.
5. Sharma OP, James DG. Did Osler's patient Hannah W, have sarcoidosis? A histological footnote. *Chest.* 1984;80: 263-4.
6. James DG, Sharma OP. Parotid gland sarcoidosis. *Sarcoidosis Vasc Diffuse Lung Dis.* 2000;17:27-32.

CHAPTER

16 Seventh Nerve Palsy (Bell's Palsy)

DEFINITION

In 1821, in a classic neurology paper submitted to the Royal Society, London, Charles Bell described 3 cases of facial nerve palsy and weakness of facial muscles; 2 cases were idiopathic and the 3rd was due to the parotid gland tumor. The unilateral palsy (paralysis) of the 7th cranial nerve is now called Bell's palsy.

HISTORY

Sir Charles Bell (1774–1842) was a Scottish anatomist, surgeon, and a member of the Royal College of Surgeons of Edinburgh. His success led to jealous opposition of local physicians and was barred from practice at the Edinburgh Royal Infirmary, the premier Scottish Medical Hospital. In 1804, he moved to London, where he set up a private surgery and school of anatomy. From 1812 to 1825, together with his brother, Bell ran the Great Windmill Street School of Anatomy, which had been founded by the great anatomist William Hunter (1718–1783). In 1824, Bell became the first professor of anatomy and surgery of the Royal College of Surgeons, London. He was made a Fellow of the Royal Society in 1826. In 1828, he helped to found the Middlesex Hospital and Medical School. Bell was knighted in 1831. He was a prolific researcher and author.

EPIDEMIOLOGY AND PATHOGENESIS

About one-half of all cases of Bell's palsy, defined as an acute peripheral facial nerve palsy, have no known cause and are classified as idiopathic. The annual incidence rate is between 20 and 32 cases per 100,000 of population.[1] There is no race, geographic, or gender predilection, but the risk is 3 times greater during pregnancy, especially in the third trimester or in the first postpartum week. Diabetes is present in about 5–10% of patient with Bell's palsy.

Herpes zoster is probably the second most common viral infection associated with facial palsy.[2] A herpes simplex-mediated viral inflammatory/immune mechanism was the subject of controversy for years, but was suspected based upon serological evidence. Polymerase chain reaction deoxyribonucleic acid testing supports the notion of axonal spread and multiplication of a reactivated neurotropic virus, leading to inflammation, demyelination, and palsy. Herpes simplex virus (HSV) activation has become widely accepted as the likely cause of Bell's palsy in most cases. HSV-1 genomes have been identified in facial nerve endoneurial fluid and auricular muscle in the patients undergoing decompression surgery for Bell's palsy, but in no controls.

Other infectious causes of Bell's palsy include cytomegalovirus, Epstein-Barr virus, adenovirus, rubella virus, mumps, influenza B, and coxsackievirus. Two cases due to Rickettsial infection have also been reported and ehrlichiosis can present as facial diplegia.

SARCOIDOSIS AND BELL'S PALSY

The unilateral 7th facial nerve is the single-most common cranial nerve lesion and the most frequent neurological manifestation of sarcoidosis. Bilateral facial involvement may occur simultaneously or sequentially. The site of the facial nerve lesion is unclear. The palsy is of peripheral or lower motor neuron type. In 1948, Colover[3] found that the facial nerve was involved in about half of the reported cases of sarcoidosis affecting the nervous system. In 1967, James and Sharma[4] reported that among 38 patients with nervous system involvement, facial nerve was affected in 25, bilaterally in 7; by contrast, other cranial nerves were affected in only 4. Nevertheless, the incidence of Bell's palsy in sarcoidosis is about 3% of the patients. Although in most cases it subsides completely leaving no sequelae, in 10–20% the lesion may remain permanent and causing facial weakness and asymmetry, hyeracusis, synkinesia, a loss of taste, and inability to produce tears.

CLINICAL FEATURES

Bell's palsy or facial paralysis is characterized by facial drooping on the affected half due to malfunction of the nerve and is typified by inability to control movement in the facial muscles. Since the 7th cranial also controls a number of other functions, such as blinking and closing the eyes, smiling, frowning, lacrimation, and salivation; these functions may be altered on the patients with Bell's palsy. Facial nerve also innervates the stapes muscles of the middle ear and carries taste sensations from the anterior two-thirds of the tongue.

PATHOGENESIS

The exact pathophysiology of Bell palsy in sarcoidosis remains unclear. The facial nerve courses through a portion of the temporal bone commonly referred to as the facial canal. One theory proposes that in sarcoidosis, granulomatous inflammation causes such edema and ischemia result in compression of the facial nerve within this bony canal. The compression can be seen in magnetic resonance imaging (MRI) scans.

DIFFERENTIAL DIAGNOSIS

The most common cause of Bell's palsy is the HSV.[2] Other viruses that have been linked to Bell's palsy include chicken-pox and shingles (herpes zoster) virus, Epstein-Bar virus, and cytomegalovirus. It is also associated with influenza or a flu-like illness, chronic middle ear infection, high blood pressure, diabetes, sarcoidosis, tumors, Lyme disease, syphilis, autoimmune diseases, demyelinating disorders, and trauma, such as skull fracture or facial injury. A family history of Bell palsy is present in about 4% of cases. Inheritance in such cases may be autosomal dominant with low penetration.

The following should always be included in differential diagnosis of facial palsy:

- Anterior circulation stroke
- Benign skull tumors
- Brainstem gliomas
- Cerebral aneurysms/intracranial hemorrhage
- Meningioma
- Meningococcal meningitis
- Neurosyphilis
- Sarcoidosis
- Tick-borne diseases
- Tuberculous meningitis
- Melkersson-rosenthal syndrome.

HEERFORDT'S SYNDROME

It is also called uveoparotid fever, Heerfordt-Mylius syndrome, Heerfordt-Waldenström syndrome, or Waldenström's uveoparotitis. It is a rare manifestation of sarcoidosis. The symptoms include inflammation of the eye (uveitis), the parotid gland swelling, fever, and in some cases, palsy of the facial nerve.

DIAGNOSIS

A detailed medical history and a thorough examination can eliminate many possible causes of the facial palsy. The joint pains, muscle weakness, or paralysis in other parts of the body point towards Lyme disease. There is no specific test for Bell's palsy, but Lyme disease, HSV, or other infection need to be excluded. A chest X-ray film is the single-most important test. In sarcoidosis, chest X-film always show bilateral hilar adenopathy with or without an infiltrate. Computed tomography scans and MRI are rarely needed, but can eliminate the structural causes compressing the facial nerve. Electromyography can confirm the presence of nerve damage and determine the severity and the extent of nerve involvement.

TREATMENT

For years, physicians have treated Bell's palsy as early as possible with corticosteroids. In addition, the detection of HSV in the endoneurial fluid of patients with Bell's palsy had led to the widespread use of antiviral agents along with corticosteroids. Most of the studies that have compared corticosteroid treatment with placebo in patients with Bell's palsy have shown significant improvement with corticosteroids. Corticosteroids decrease the incidence of permanent facial paralysis. Sullivan et al. showed that combining acyclovir with corticosteroids produced no extra benefit. Treatment is a matter of controversy.[5] In patients presenting with incomplete facial palsy, where the prognosis for recovery is very good, treatment is unnecessary. The Copenhagen Facial Nerve Study examined 2,570 cases of peripheral facial nerve palsy over a period of 25 year.[6] There were 1,701 cases of Bell's palsy and 869 of non-Bell's palsy. Of the total patient population, 116 had herpes zoster, 76 had diabetes, 46 were pregnant, and 169 were neonates. A total of 38 different etiologies were observed. The initial examination revealed 30% incomplete and 70% complete palsies. Follow-up showed that in 85% of patients, function was returned within 3 weeks and in the remaining 15% after 3–5 months.

However, patients presenting with complete paralysis, marked by an inability to close the eyes and mouth on the involved side, are usually treated with corticosteroids. Rationale for early and aggressive treatment is based on the observation of the presence of facial nerve swelling. Edema may be secondary to inflammation, granulomas formation in the nerve wall, or ischemia. Edema can be demonstrated by MRI in 9–23 days after the onset of Bells' palsy. Surgical procedures to decompress the facial nerve have not been proven beneficial. Several procedures aimed at protecting the cornea from exposure and achieving facial symmetry is required in selected cases. These procedures may reduce the need for constant use of lubrication drops or ointments, improve cosmetic appearance, and help to preserve vision on the affected side.

CASE STUDY

A 49-year-old female patient was referred to an otorhinolaryngology clinic due to left-sided hearing loss and peripheral facial nerve paralysis that occurred suddenly. Two months earlier, she complained of unilateral tinnitus, fatigue, and occasional headaches. She was treated in a local hospital for the diagnosis of serous otitis media where she underwent paracentesis and prolonged medical therapy, including antibiotics and nasal topical decongestants (Figure 16-1).

On otoscopic examination, the left tympanic membrane was hyperemic and perforated due to previous paracentesis. There were no vestibular symptoms and none were related to her nose and throat. The patient had left facial paralysis (VI grade in House-Brackman Facial Paralysis Scale). Audiometric evaluation revealed mixed-type hearing loss on the left side.

Computed tomography of the temporal bone was performed and revealed soft tissue density in mastoid cells on the left side which extended to the tympanic cavity (Figure 16-2).

Based on these findings, an explorative surgery was performed on the left ear. At open tympanoplasty, pale pink granular mass was seen filling mastoid cells and extending into the aditus and toward the epitympanum and tegmen tympani. After the removal of granulation tissue, the partial facial decompression was performed due to suprastapedial herniation of the nerve. Histopathologic examination showed several small granulomas with epitheloid cells surrounded by rim of lymphocytes, finding typical for sarcoidosis. Acid-fast bacilli were not observed. The facial paralysis improved immediately after the surgery (Grade I/II in House-Brackman Facial Paralysis Scale). Chest X-ray represented bilateral hilar adenopathy without parenchymal lesions. She was treated with steroid therapy. She has completely recovered.

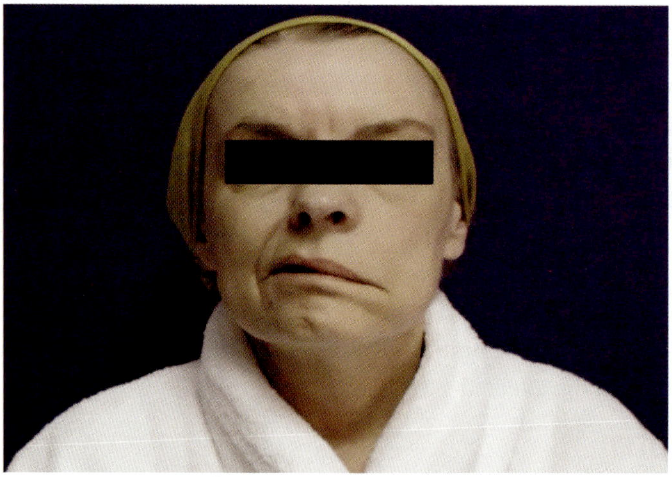

Figure 16-1 A 49-year-old female patient with left-sided hearing loss and peripheral facial nerve paralysis.

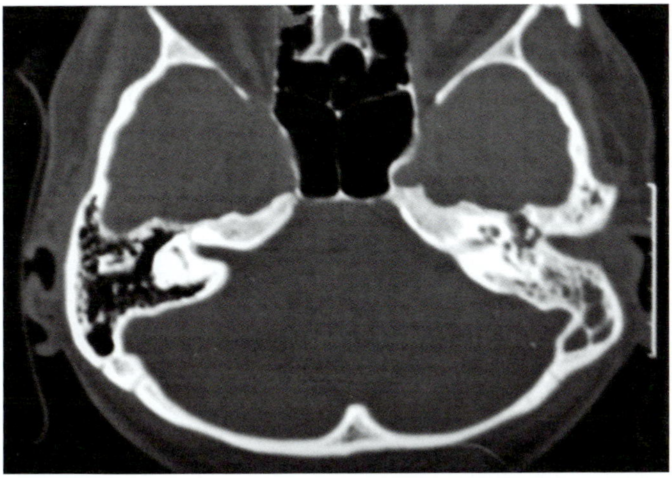

Figure 16-2 Axial section of computed tomographic scan showing middle ear and mastoid soft tissue mass due to sarcoid granulomas. *Courtesy:* Professor Nenad Arsovic. Otorynolaryngology Clinic, Clinical Center Belgrade, Serbia.

REFERENCES

1. Gilden DH, Tyler KL. Bell's palsy--is glucocorticoid treatment enough? *N Engl J Med.* 2007;357:1653-5.
2. Schirm J, Mulkens PS. Bell's palsy and herpes simplex virus. *APMIS.* 1997;105:815-23.
3. Colover J. Sarcoidosis with involvement of the nervous system. *Brain.* 1948;71;451-75.
4. James DG, Sharma OP. Neurosarcoidosis. *Proc R Soc Med.* 1967;60:1169-70.
5. Sullivan FM, Swan IR, Donnan PT, Morrison JM, Smith BH, McKinstry B, et al. Early treatment with prednisolone or acyclovir in Bell's palsy. *N Engl J Med.* 2007;357:1598-607.
6. Peitersen E. Bell's palsy: the spontaneous course of 2,500 peripheral facial nerve palsies of different etiologies. *Acta Otolaryngol Suppl.* 2002;4-30.

CHAPTER
17 Hepatic Granulomas and Isolated Serum Alkaline Phosphatase Level

DEFINITION

Sheila Sherlock wrote, "All granulomas represent a response to antigenic stimuli. The liver is particularly involved because of the very large number of sinusoidal cells. These include the Kupffer cells which endocytose old cells, foreign particles, tumor cells, bacteria, yeasts, viruses, and parasites. It is not surprising that the liver is involved almost in all types of granulomas".[1]

HISTORY

Sheila Sherlock (1918–2001) graduated from Edinburgh University with a gold medal. She went to the Hammersmith Hospital where she established the world's first liver disease unit. Thriving on the vibrant research atmosphere, she produced an array of landmark studies on liver disease. With John Guy Scadding, she published the first paper on the role of liver biopsy in diagnosing sarcoidosis. The procedure was commonly used for decades before it lost ground to transbronchial lung biopsy. Sherlock's textbook, "Diseases of the Liver and Biliary" system ran in 11 editions in her lifetime and was translated into German, Japanese, Greek, Italian, Russian, Spanish, and Portuguese. In 1978, she was made Dame of the British Empire.[2]

John Guyet Scadding (1907–1999), father of respiratory medicine in Britain, was one of the most brilliant physicians of his generation. He was only 27 years old when he was appointed as consultant physician at the British (now Royal) Postgraduate Medical School and Hammersmith Hospital. His publications covered many aspects of respiratory medicine, but he is best remembered for his seminal work on sarcoidosis and interstitial pulmonary fibrosis.

INCIDENCE

Hepatic granulomas are found in 4–10% of needle liver biopsies. In 10%, no cause is found even after an extensive search, including specific stains and culture for various organisms, immunological tests for autoimmune reactions, and examination of the tissue under polarizing light to exclude foreign particles.

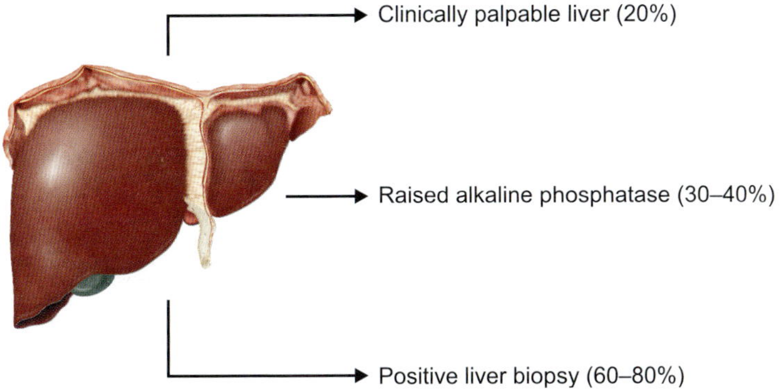

Figure 17-1 Liver involvement in sarcoidosis (percentage of patients).

Sherlock and Scadding performed liver biopsies in 73 patients with sarcoidosis and found granulomas in 48 (68%); when chest X-ray showed only bilateral hilar adenopathy (stage I), 87% were positive; when there was bilateral hilar adenopathy and infiltration (stage II), 67% were positive; and when chest X-ray showed only infiltration (stage III), 59% were positive.[3] Klatskin reported an even higher incidence of 94%.[4]

CLINICAL PICTURE

The liver is frequently affected in sarcoidosis, but the granulomatous inflammation is often asymptomatic. Overt hepatic insufficiency and failure are rare. The liver is palpable in 20% of the patients, alkaline phosphatase is elevated in 30–40%, and 60–80% of the patients with sarcoidosis have granulomas in liver biopsy specimens (Figure 17-1).

HISTOLOGY

Hepatic granulomas vary between 50 and 500 μm in diameter. Serial sections must be cut if granulomas are to be found. Granulomas are found everywhere in the liver, but most frequently near portal tracts. They are well formed, compact, sharply defined, randomly distributed, and surrounded by normal hepatic parenchymal tissue (Figure 17-2). In sarcoidosis, granulomas are repetitively monotonous being in the same stage of development. Multinucleated giant cells may be present, but asteroid and Schaumann inclusions are rare. The granulomas are randomly distributed and heal with little or no fibrosis.

DIFFERENTIAL DIAGNOSIS

There are many causes of hepatic granulomas (Table 17-1). Necrotizing or caseating granulomas have a necrotic center and a histiocytic rim with palisading pattern.

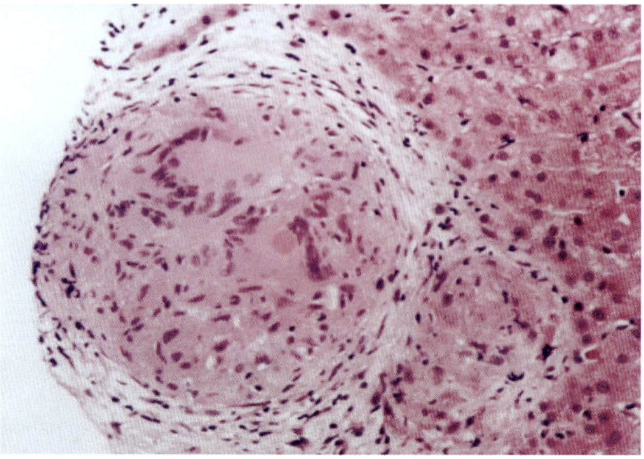

Figure 17-2 Sarcoid granuloma of the liver. Typical appearance with multinuclear giant cells.

Table 17-1 Causes and Evaluation of Hepatic Granuloma

Disease	*Evaluation*
Sarcoidosis	Chest X-ray, HRCT, ACE, BAL, transbronchial biopsy, and gallium scan
Tuberculosis	Chest X-ray, sputum examination, tuberculin test, BAL, and QFT test
Coccidioidomycosis	History of being in endemic zone, and complement-fixation test
Histoplasmosis	Chest X-ray
Brucellosis	History, blood culture, and agglutinin titer
Primary biliary cirrhosis	Mitochondrial antibody
Syphilis	Treponema test
Leprosy	History and lepromin test
Berylliosis	History of exposure and chest X-ray
Lymphoma	Chest X-ray, B-symptoms, and biopsy of the lymph node
Q-fever	History and antibodies
AIDS	Poorly formed granulomas, acid-fast and fungal stains

HRCT, high resolution computed tomography; ACE, angiotensin converting enzyme; BAL, broncho-alveolar lavage; QFT, QuantiFERON; AIDS, acquired immunodeficiency disease.

Fibrosis is variable. Such granulomas are often associated with tuberculosis, fungi, and rarely with Hodgkin's lymphoma.

In an asymptomatic patient with or without any symptoms and signs of hepatic or extrahepatic disease, the granulomas should be ignored, but the patient should be observed yearly for 3–4 years.

TREATMENT

The treatment of hepatic sarcoidosis depends upon the clinical manifestations of the disease. As mentioned above, the majority of patients are asymptomatic,

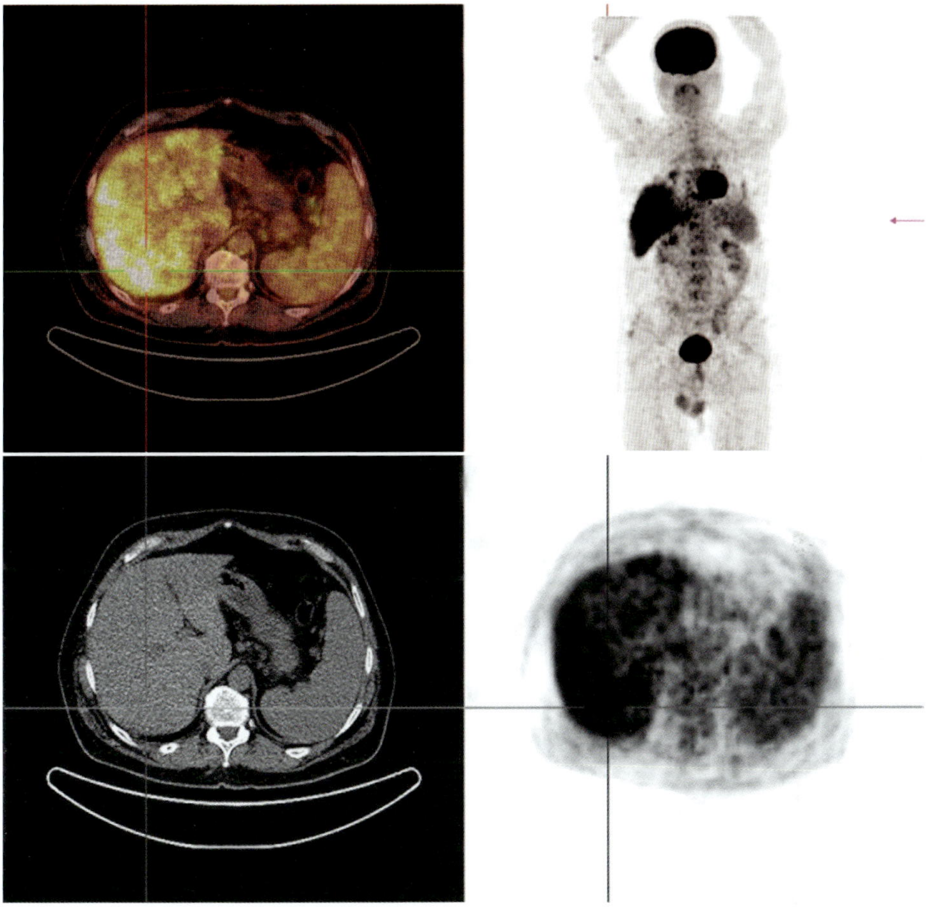

Figure 17-3 and 4 18-fluorodeoxyglucose positron emission tomography in patient with lung and liver sarcoidosis. In the vast majority of patients with sarcoidosis, the diagnosis is available by biopsy of a wide variety of organs. If the diagnosis is to be pursued, whole-body 18-fluorodeoxyglucose positron emission tomography (18FDG PET) scan imaging may uncover an occult diagnostic site or multiple organ involvement. This patient already had biopsy positive lung sarcoidosis. His liver enzymes were within normal values, alkaline phosphatase too. 18FDG PET scan, however, revealed active disease of the liver. Biopsy confirmed hepatic sarcoid granulomas. *Courtesy:* Professor Dragana Sobic-Saranovic. National PET Scan Center, Clinical Center Belgrade, Serbia.

and thus do not require specific treatment. Whether corticosteroids could prevent hepatic disease progression or the development of complications is unproven and, therefore, not recommended for hepatic disease alone. In patients with severe cholestasis or portal hypertension and constitutional symptoms, a short course of corticosteroids can be considered to see if the patient has a favorable response. Unless the patient has severe liver dysfunction, it is worthwhile to wait and follow the patient clinically and check liver functions periodically. If the treatment is required then prednisone should be given, but the benefits of long-term treatment must be balanced against side effects. Chloroquine is an effective alternative in patients who develop devastating side effects of corticosteroids.[5]

CASE STUDY

In 1980, during a pre-employment health evaluation, this 49-year-old, asymptomatic, African-American woman was found to have a bilateral hilar adenopathy on a chest X-ray film, an elevated serum alkaline level, and a normal serum angiotensin converting level. Liver biopsy showed noncaseating granulomas. Because she was symptomatic and has normal serum glutamic oxaloacetic transaminase and serum glutamic pyruvate transaminase, no treatment was given for her isolated alkaline phosphatase elevation. For 14 years, she remained asymptomatic and serum alkaline showed spontaneous variations. In 1994, liver biopsy was repeated which showed a few smaller noncaseating granulomas (Figure 17-2).

REFERENCES

1. Sherlock S, Dooley J. Disease of the liver and gall bladder. London: Blackwell; 2001.
2. Sharma OP. Prof: the life of Sheila Sherlock: the Liver Queen. London: Royal College of Physicians of London; 2007.
3. Scadding JG. Sarcoidosis. London: Eyre and Spottiswoode; 1967.
4. Klatskin G. Hepatic granulomata: problems in interpretation. *Mt Sinai J Med.* 1977;4 4: 798-812.
5. Vatti R, Sharma OP. Liver involvement in sarcoidosis: role of therapy in selected cases. *Sarcoidosis Vasc Diffuse Lung Dis.* 1997;14:73-6.

CHAPTER

18 Enlarged Spleen

ANATOMY

The spleen in healthy adult humans is approximately 11 cm in length and weighs between 150 and 250 g. About the size of a clenched fist, it lies in the left upper quadrant of the abdomen, beneath the 9th to the 12th thoracic ribs.

As a part of the spleen mononuclear phagocyte system, it metabolizes hemoglobin removed from dead erythrocytes. It synthesizes antibodies in its white pulp and removes antibody-coated bacteria. Within the red pulp, the spleen has about half of the body's monocytes. These monocytes move to injured tissue and turn into dendritic cells and macrophages. The spleen is the center of activity of the reticuloendothelial system; its absence can predispose to certain infections.

INCIDENCE

The spleen must double in size before it can be palpated beyond the costal margin. The term massive splenomegaly denotes splenic weight more than 1,000 g or 4–6 times the normal weight. Asymptomatic splenic involvement is common in sarcoidosis. At autopsy, splenic granulomas are seen in 38–77% of sarcoidosis patients.[1] Longcope and Freiman reported that spleen was enlarged in 65% of the autopsied subjects with sarcoidosis.[2] Selroos and Koievunen performed needle aspiration biopsies in 312 Finnish patients and found granulomas in 184 (53%).[3] Turiaf and Battesti carried out celiac arteriography in 28 sarcoidosis patients, the spleen was enlarged in 15 (53%).[4] Using ultrasound examination, splenomegaly was detected in 22 of 108 (20.03%) patients at the Clinical Center of Serbia, Belgrade.[5]

CLINICAL FEATURES

Symptoms of splenic infiltration occur in less than 2% of patients and are usually limited to those with massive splenomegaly (Figure 18-1). Fever, early satiety, weight loss, and left upper quadrant fullness and ache are the common symptoms. Occasionally, severe pain due to splenic infarct secondary to compression may be the initial clinical symptom. Massive splenomegaly may cause anemia, leucopenia

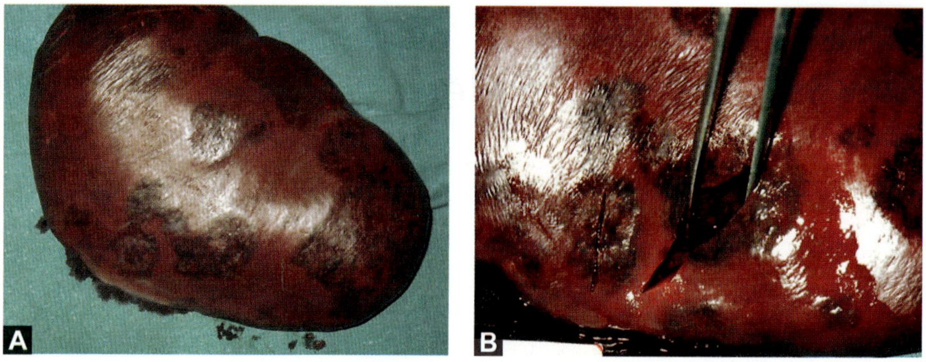

Figure 18-1 Splenomegaly in sarcoidosis. The weight of a normal spleen is approximately 150–250 g. This spleen after splenectomy weighted 3 kg. *Courtesy* Professor Vesna Skodric-Trifunovic, from the Clinic of Pulmonary Diseases, Clinical center Belgrade, Serbia, who diagnosed and treated the patient.

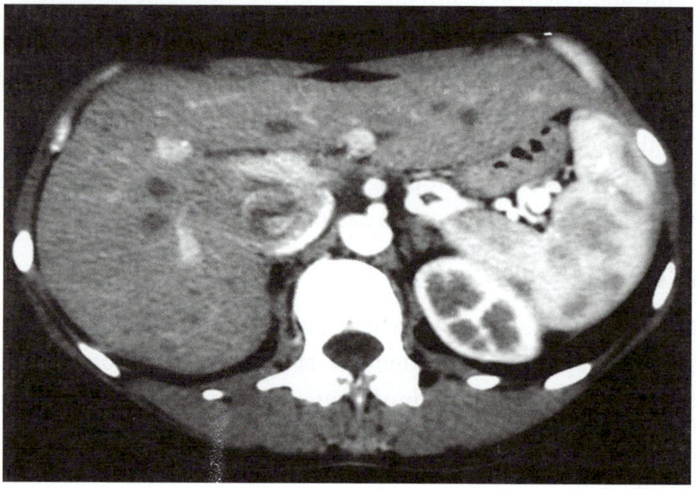

Figure 18-2 Computed tomography examination of the spleen. *Courtesy* Professor Vesna Skodric-Trifunovic, from the Clinic of Pulmonary Diseases, Clinical center Belgrade, Serbia, who diagnosed and treated the patient, *with permission*.

and thrombocytopenia, fatigue, and petechiae. These patients tend to have high levels of serum angiotensin converting enzyme levels.

INVESTIGATIONS

On abdominal computed tomographic examination, the spleen may appear as a homogenous density (Figure 18-2). If the granulomas fuse together, they form multiple low attenuation nodular densities. In a study of 32 sarcoidosis patients, multiple attenuation areas were present in all.

Hypermetabolic spleen lesions with a maximal standardized uptake value (SUV) of 15.8. Fluorodeoxyglucose positron emission tomography (FDG PET) scan imaging is expensive and not available to all patients with sarcoidosis; however, a positive FDG PET scan finding is not a diagnosis of sarcoidosis. Positive scan findings occur in patients with other granulomatous diseases, infections, and neoplasms. Patients with sarcoidosis may have comorbid FDG PET scan positive disease. The clinician must take that into consideration when accepting positive findings of an FDG PET scan of a lesion as being due to a tumor (Figure 18-3).

TREATMENT

The primary treatment for symptomatic splenomegaly in sarcoidosis is corticosteroids (Figure 18-4). Methotrexate and azthioprine are used in patients refractory or intolerant to corticosteroids. Splenectomy may become necessary in patients with massive splenomegaly as a precaution against splenic rupture, severe hypersplenism unresponsive to medical treatment, and need for excluding lymphoma or malignancy.

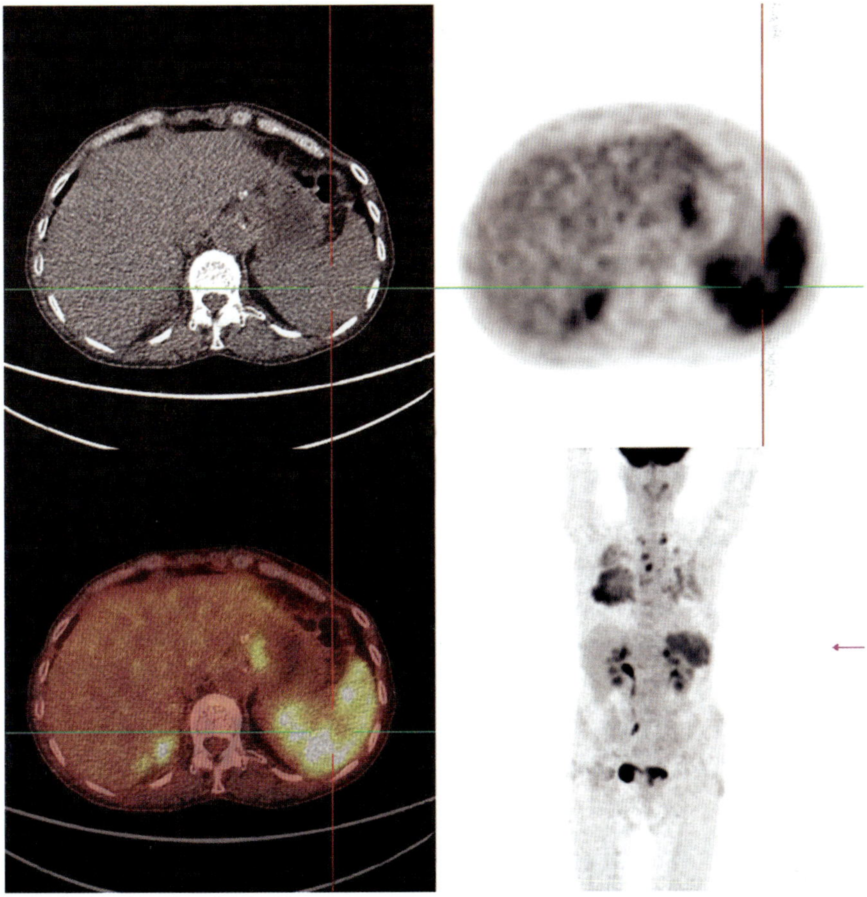

Figure 18-3 The whole-body fluorodeoxyglucose positron emission tomography scan imaging may uncover an occult diagnostic site or multiple organ involvement.

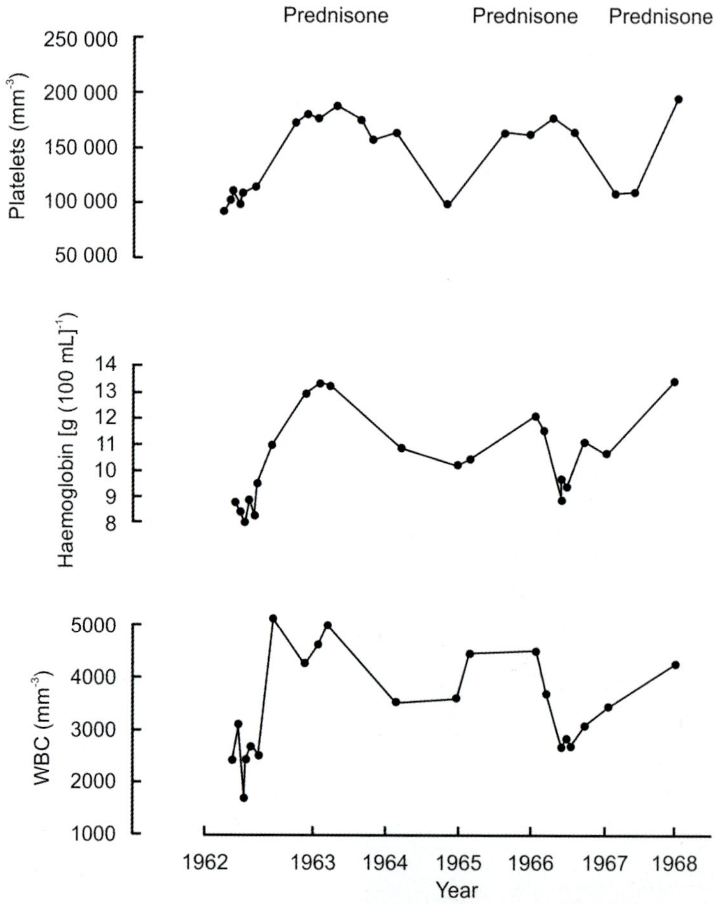

Figure 18-4 Anemia, leucopenia, and thrombocytopenia caused by hypersplenism responded nicely to prednisone treatment. WBC, white blood cell. *Source:* Sharma OP. Sarcoidosis: Clinical Management. London: Butterworths; 1984. p. 84.

REFERENCES

1. Sharma OP, Vucinic V, James DG. Splenectomy in sarcoidosis: indications, complications, and long-term follow-up. *Sarcoidosis Vasc Diffuse Lung Dis.* 2002;19:66-70.
2. Longcope W, Freiman DG. A study of sarcoidosis based on a combined investigation of 160 cases including 30 autopsies from the Johns Hopkins Hospital and Massachusetts General Hospital. *Medicine (Baltimore).* 1952;31:1-132.
3. Selroos O, Koivunen E. Usefulness of fine aspiration needle biopsy of spleen in sarcoidosis. *Chest.* 1983;83:193-5.
4. Turiaf J, Battesti J, Helenon C. Selective arteriography of the celiac artery in patients with thoracic sarcoidosis. *Ann N Y Acad Sci.* 1976;278:433-8.
5. Skodric V, Radivojevic S, Stevic R. The frequency of splenomegaly in sarcoid patients. *Sarcoidosis Vasc Diffuse Lung Dis.* 2001;18:54.

CHAPTER

19 Cardiac Manifestations of Sarcoidosis

INTRODUCTION

Bernstein and associates were the first group to describe cardiac sarcoidosis in 1929.[1] Hageman and Wurm estimated cardiac involvement in sarcoidosis to be 5%.[2] A report from John Hopkins showed that 27% of sarcoid patients have myocardial granulomas.[3]

CLINICAL FEATURES

Most patients are asymptomatic and those that are symptomatic may have varying manifestations of the disease, depending on the location and extent of involvement of the cardiac tissue. The myocardial conduction system is highly susceptible to sarcoid granulomas. There may be total destruction of the sinoatrial node or atrioventricular node. Fleming found complete heart block to be the most common mode of presentation in cardiac sarcoid patients. Complete heart block tends to occur at a younger age in sarcoidosis patients than in those with acquired heart block. To a lesser degree, patients may have first-degree heart block that may progress to complete heart block.[4]

Ventricular arrhythmias, such as ventricular tachycardia or premature ventricular beats are the second most common forms of presentation. The arrhythmias arise due to the granulomas in the ventricular myocardium disrupting conduction. This is a cause for concern as it is a cause of sudden death in these patients. In fact, sudden cardiac death due to ventricular tachycardia or fibrillation is responsible for 30–65% of deaths in sarcoidosis. In contrast, supraventricular arrhythmias are rare compared to ventricular arrhythmias.

Congestive heart failure is not an uncommon finding, usually occurring after the myocardial tissue has been over burdened with sarcoid granulomas. Both systolic and diastolic dysfunction may occur. Cardiomegaly is a rare finding in cardiac sarcoidosis. The cause of death is estimated to be 25% of these patients, making it the second most common cause of death in patients with cardiac sarcoidosis.

Valvular dysfunction may be another presenting problem for patients. Mitral incompetence due to papillary muscle involvement may occur, leading to eventual pulmonary hypertension, and rarely requiring valve replacement. Calcified mitral valve leading to mitral stenosis is also a known complication in the setting of hypercalcemia in sarcoidosis patients. Tricuspid regurgitation due to sarcoid infiltration has been reported, although it is very rare.

Other rare cardiac entities include a phenomenon termed simulated myocardial infarct, in which sarcoidosis may mimic an infarct by producing classic clinical symptoms and electrocardiogram findings. Rarely, pericarditis may occur due to cardiac sarcoidosis. Sarcoidosis may cause right heart failure, secondary to pulmonary hypertension in fibrotic lung disease.[5-12]

DIAGNOSIS

Cardiac involvement is common in patients with sarcoidosis, but is often clinically silent. The diagnosis of cardiac sarcoidosis should be suspected in young patients with unexplained sustained second or third degree atrioventricular block, in patients with sustained monomorphic ventricular tachycardia and dilated cardiomyopathy, and in patients with a histologic proved sarcoidosis who develop arrhythmias and heart failure. Initial history and physical examination evaluation should be augmented by electrocardiography, Holter monitoring, and echocardiography.

Cardiovascular magnetic resonance imaging (Figures 19-1 and 19-2) or fluorodeoxyglucose positron emission positron with myocardial perfusion imaging are the most sensitive tests for diagnosis of sarcoidosis. Coronary angiography is indicated to exclude coronary vascular disease. Electrophysiologic testing is suggested in patients with symptoms (palpitations, syncope, and presyncope) or nonsustained

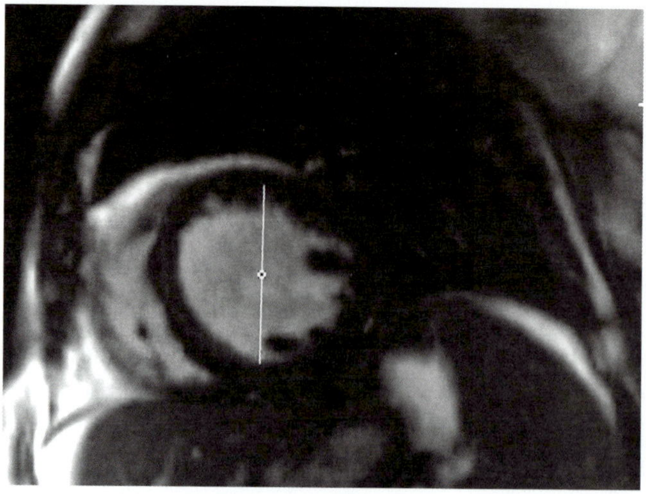

Figure 19-1 Cardiovascular magnetic resonance imaging in sarcoidosis patient with rhythm disorders (ventricular tachycardia).

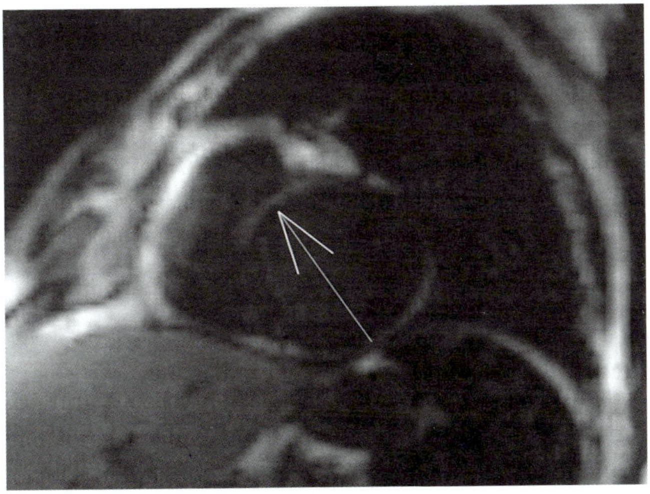

Figure 19-2 Cardiovascular magnetic resonance after contrast application. Arrow pointing out possible granuloma location. Patient had biopsy-positive lung sarcoidosis.

ventricular arrhythmias. Endomyocardial biopsy is required only if the patient has no histologic confirmation from an extracardiac site.

PROGNOSIS

Implantable cardioverter defibrillator therapy is indicated in patients with refractory ventricular tachyarrhythmias and in selected patients and New York Heart Association class II to III heart failure with a left ventricular ejection fraction ≤35%. The prognosis of cardiac sarcoidosis is not well defined but appears to be poor in those with symptomatic cardiac involvement. While patients with asymptomatic cardiac sarcoidosis generally have a more benign course, sudden death can occur as an initial clinical manifestation of disease.

REFERENCES

1. Bernstein M, Konzelmann FW, Sidlick DM. Boeck's sarcoid: report of case with visceral involvement. *Arch Intern Med.* 1929;44:721-34.
2. Hageman GJ, Wurm K. [Be alert to heart involvement in sarcoidosis]. *Med Klin.* 1980; 75:655-9.
3. Silverman KJ, Hutchins GM, Bulkley BH. Cardiac sarcoidosis: a clinicopathological study of 84 in selected patients with systemic sarcoidosis. *Circulation.* 1978;58:1204-11.
4. Fleming HA. Cardiac sarcoidosis. *Clin Dermatol.* 1986;4:143-9.
5. Dubrey SW, Falk RH. Diagnosis and management of cardiac sarcoidosis. *Prog Cardiovasc Dis.* 2010;52:336-46.
6. Pierre-Louis B, Prasad A, Frishman WH. Cardiac manifestations of sarcoidosis and therapeutic options. *Cardiol Rev.* 2009;17:153-8.
7. Chapelon-Abric C, de Zuttere D, Duhaut P, Veyssier P, Wechsler B, Huong DL, et al. Cardiac sarcoidosis: a retrospective study of 41 cases. *Medicine (Baltimore).* 2004;83: 315-34.

8. Cheong BY, Muthupillai R, Nemeth M, Lambert B, Dees D, Huber S, et al. The utility of delayed-enhancement magnetic resonance imaging for identifying nonischemic myocardial fibrosis in asymptomatic patients with biopsy-proven systemic sarcoidosis. *Sarcoidosis Vasc Diffuse Lung Dis.* 2009;26:39-46.
9. Nomura S, Funabashi N, Tsubura M, Uehara M, Shiina Y, Daimon M, et al. Cardiac sarcoidosis evaluated by multimodality imaging. *Int J Cardiol.* 2011;150:e81-4.
10. Kudoh H, Fujiwara S, Shiotani H, Kawai H, Hirata K. Myocardial washout of 99m Tc-tetrofosmin and response to steroid therapy in patients with cardiac sarcoidosis. *Ann Nucl Med.* 2010;24:379-85.
11. Sharma S. Cardiac imaging in myocardial sarcoidosis and other cardiomyopathies. *Curr Opin Pulm Med.* 2009;15:507-12.
12. Sharma PS, Lubahn JG, Donsky AS, Yoon AD, Carry MM, Grayburn PA, et al. Diagnosing cardiac sarcoidosis clinically without tissue confirmation. *Proc (Bayl Univ Med Cent).* 2009;22:236-8.
13. Sharma OP, Maheshwari A, Thaker K. Myocardial sarcoidosis. *Chest.* 1993;103:253-8.

CHAPTER

20 Neurosarcoidosis

INTRODUCTION

Clinically recognizable involvement of the central nervous system (CNS) occurs in 2–7% of patients with sarcoidosis. Noncaseating sarcoid granulomas have been observed in up to 14% of sarcoid patients at necropsy. An unequivocal diagnosis of neurosarcoidosis requires a compatible clinical or radiological picture and histologic confirmation of noncaseating granulomas. Because of the relative inaccessibility and risk of biopsies of CNS lesions, a diagnosis of neurosarcoidosis can be presumed in patients with known sarcoidosis at other sites and compatible magnetic resonance image (MRI) scans. Gallium 67-scans or chest computed tomography scans may be helpful in establishing involvement at extraneural sites. Serial MRI scans can be performed to determine therapeutic efficacy. Therapeutic failure warrants a more aggressive diagnostic approach, which includes biopsies of CNS lesions.

Neurologic manifestations include:

- Cranial nerve involvement
- Peripheral neuropathy (alone or with cranial nerve palsies)
- Seizures
- Meningitis
- Space occupying lesions
- Hypothalamic and pituitary gland sarcoidosis
- Cerebellar ataxia
- Spinal cord involvement
- Psychiatric symptoms.

CRANIAL NERVE INVOLVEMENT

Any cranial nerve can be affected, although the most frequently affected is the seventh, sometimes in association with uveitis and parotitis (uveoparotid fever), but usually alone, thus suggesting Bell palsy (see chapter 16). Facial weakness can be bilateral and either simultaneous or sequential, and can recur after recovery. It is unilateral in 65% and bilateral in 35%. The mechanism of facial nerve involvement in sarcoidosis remains unclear. Some authors consider facial palsy to be a type of "cranial polyneuritis."

Optic nerve involvement causes papillitis or retrobulbar neuritis and eventually optic atrophy. Trigeminal nerve involvement causes either sensory loss or neuralgia, and eighth cranial nerve lesions produce auditory and vestibular symptoms.[1-7]

PAPILLEDEMA

Papilledema was observed in 18% in one series of the patients with neurosarcoidosis.[7] The diagnosis of neurosarcoidosis should be entertained in young adults, particularly women of childbearing age, with rapidly developing papilledema associated with the seventh or other cranial nerve palsies.

PERIPHERAL NEUROPATHY

The overall incidence of peripheral neuropathy is unknown. Peripheral nerve involvement may occur either alone or in association with other cranial nerve palsies, although the latter occurrence is infrequent. All types of neuropathy—mononeuritis, polyneuritis, Landry's, or Guillain-Barre syndrome—have been described, but the pathogenesis of neuropathy is not well defined.[7]

Manifestations of peripheral neuropathy in sarcoid patients include paresthesia, root pains, weakness and wasting of muscles, absence or depression of tendon reflexes, and neuralgia (either symmetric or asymmetric).[7,8]

Sarcoid patients without neurologic symptoms show low amplitude of evoked sensory potentials in one or more nerves, suggesting that subclinical involvement of nerves may be common in sarcoidosis.

SEIZURES

Seizures occur in 5–22% of patients with neurosarcoidosis and indicate chronicity and poor prognosis.[7,8]

MENINGITIS

Meningeal symptoms occur in 3–26% of patients with neurosarcoidosis. Symptoms and signs include fever, headache, and neck rigidity.[8,9] Acute meningitis responds to corticosteroids, while chronic meningitis with multiple remissions and exacerbations requires long-term therapy.

HYDROCEPHALUS

Hydrocephalus, an undesirable complication in sarcoidosis, is rare (Figures 20-1 and 20-2).[8]

SPACE OCCUPYING LESIONS

Localized granulomatous mass lesions have been found in every part of the CNS, including the floor of the third ventricle, the occipital, frontal and temporal lobes, the optic chiasma, the basal ganglion, and the cerebellum (Figure 20-3). Clinical

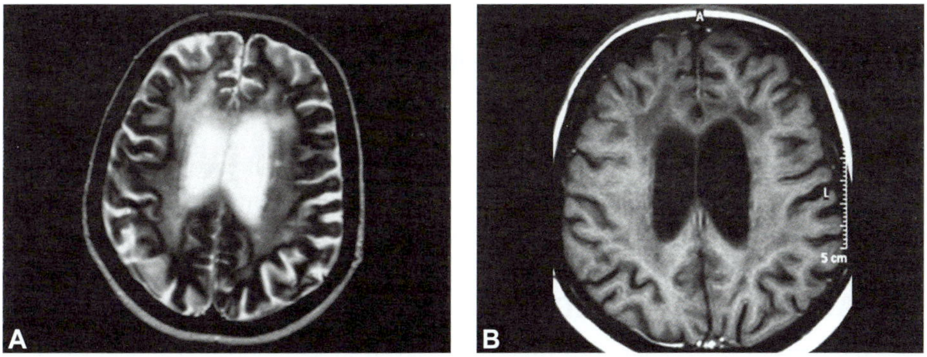

Figure 20-1 Hydrocephalus in sarcoidosis. This patient had biopsy positive pulmonary sarcoidosis. Cerebrospinal fluid (CSF) analyses: angiotensin converting enzyme (ACE) levels of 15 U/L.

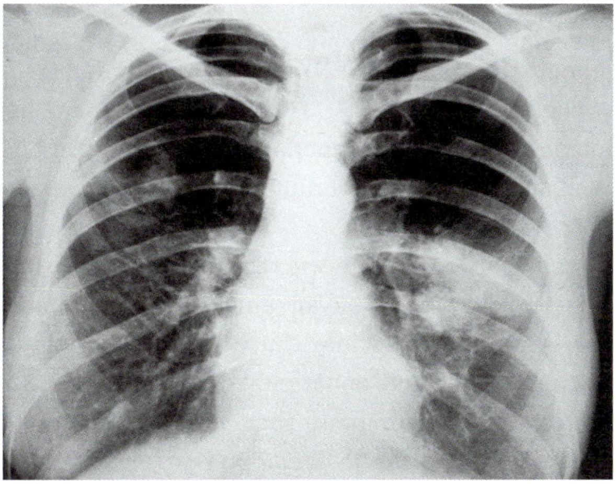

Figure 20-2 Chest X-ray of the same patient presenting adenopathy with parenchymal lesions.

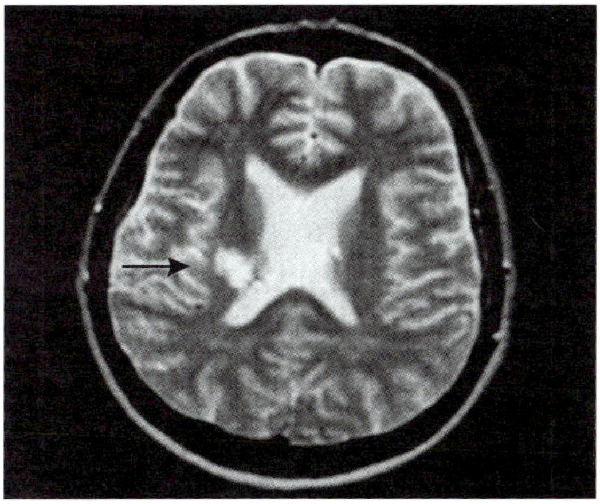

Figure 20-3 Space occupying lesion in patient with neurosarcoidosis (arrow).

symptoms are similar to any space-occupying mass—headaches, lethargy, seizures, diminution of visual acuity, papilledema, and optic atrophy.[7]

HYPOTHALAMIC AND PITUITARY GLAND SARCOIDOSIS

Granulomatous involvement of the base of the brain is well-recognized. Diabetes insipidus is a common presentation, while hyperprolactinemia and galactorrhea-amenorrhea syndrome are less common.[7,8]

SPINAL CORD IN SARCOIDOSIS

Any segment of the spinal cord may be involved in sarcoidosis. Clinical signs of spinal cord dysfunction include paraparesis, tetraparesis, back and leg pains, and incontinence; hemiparesis is less common.[8]

SMALL FIBER NEUROPATHY

Recently, small fiber neuropathy (SFN) was demonstrated in sarcoidosis and appeared to be relatively frequent.[10-12] However, as standard nerve conduction tests evaluate only large nerve fiber function and quantitative techniques for the assessment of small nerve fibers are not routinely applied, the diagnosis of SFN can easily be missed.

SFN has only relatively recently been recognized as a distinct entity. If not recognized, these symptoms may be an enigma to both patient and doctor. Recognition of SFN is important as it may cause disabling symptoms. SFN may also involve autonomic nerve fibers and, apparently, cardiac sympathetic denervation.[13]

Whether life-threatening symptoms, such as cardiac arrhythmias occur in sarcoidosis when cardiac autonomic denervation is involved requires further study. SFN may also cause restless leg syndrome (RLS).[14] RLS and periodic limb movement disorder (PLMD) are frequently associated and related to sleep disturbances. PLMD and RLS have been found to be present in sarcoidosis.[15,16]

PSYCHIATRIC SYMPTOMS

Granulomatous infiltration of the CNS may produce a wide variety of mental symptoms. In a patient with multisystemic sarcoidosis and unexplained mental deterioration, aggressive evaluation of the CNS is indicated. Symptoms may respond to corticoid therapy. A subset of sarcoidosis patients present with mild amnesic problems, without objective deterioration or neurological deficit. This might be related to fatigue and concentration problems.[17,18]

DIAGNOSIS OF NEUROSARCOIDOSIS

Three possible clinical situations can be distinguished in patients with neuro-sarcoidosis:

1. Patients with neurological features and histologically confirmed active systemic sarcoidosis.
2. Patients with neurological features and a history of sarcoidosis without any evidence of activity.
3. Patients with neurological features without a history of or any evidence of systemic sarcoidosis.

In patients with neurological features and histologically confirmed active systemic sarcoidosis, neurological symptoms are most probably related to systemic sarcoidosis and there is justification in starting therapy.[8] However, when treatment fails, the diagnosis should be reassessed and an attempt made to obtain biopsy specimens in order to establish the correct diagnosis.

In patients with a history of sarcoidosis who present with neurological symptoms, neurosarcoidosis will be considered early in the differential diagnosis. The need for biopsy is crucial in such a situation.

In patients with neurological features without a history of or any evidence of systemic sarcoidosis, neurosarcoidosis will rarely be considered at an early stage. In these cases, neurosarcoidosis remains one of the more challenging diagnostic problems.[19]

A prior history of sarcoidosis does not necessarily mean that any new problem of the patient is automatically attributable to sarcoidosis. The approach in a patient with a prior history of sarcoidosis without evidence of current active disease should be the same as in a patient without a history of sarcoidosis.

Whole-body gallium scanning or fluorodeoxyglucose positron emission tomography (PET) can be utilized in finding other suitable sites for biopsy (Figure 20-5).[20,21]

If no evidence of systemic sarcoidosis is found, but a CNS biopsy reveals a sarcoid-like granulomatous reaction, there should be awareness of the distinction between systemic neurosarcoidosis and a local (neurological) sarcoid-like reaction, particularly related to an old scar or a helminthic reaction.[16]

Imaging Techniques in Neurosarcoidosis

Both CT and MRI are useful in diagnosis of neurological sarcoidosis. Contrast enhanced CT may detect meningeal disease, parenchymal mass lesions, nodules or plaques, periventricular white matter lesions, and obstructive/communicating hydrocephalus.

Abnormalities on CT are nonspecific, as similar lesions may be observed in carcinomatous, bacterial, or fungal meningitis. CT may be normal in up to 30% of patients with neurosarcoidosis, especially when lesions are confined to the cranial or peripheral nerves or brainstem.[22] MRI is superior to CT in visualizing sarcoid lesions in parenchyma, periventricular white matter, hypothalamus, and spinal cord.[20,23]

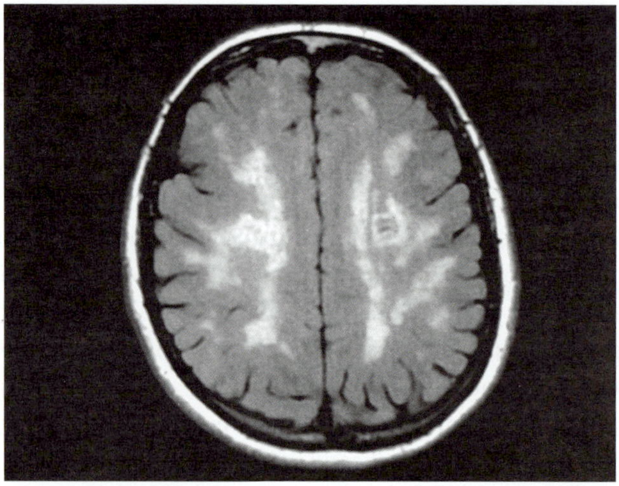

Figure 20-4 Magnetic resonance of the brain shows hyper intense lesions of the white matter, bilateral, occipital, and parietal lobes.

Gadolinium-enhanced MRI is the preferred and the most useful test in assessing the extent and following the course of CNS sarcoidosis (Figure 20-4). A normal MRI does not exclude neurosarcoidosis especially in patients with only cranial neuropathies or receiving corticosteroids.[20-24] Unenhanced MRI imaging is unsatisfactory because of the poor contrast among bone, cerebrospinal fluid (CSF), and meninges on both T helper (Th)1 and Th2 weighted series.[24,25]

Multifocal periventricular and subcortical white matter abnormalities, clustered near regions of meningeal enhancement, are characteristic of neurosarcoidosis.

Cerebrospinal Fluid in Neurosarcoidosis

Routine CSF abnormalities are usually nonspecific and include mild pleocytosis, increased protein content, and sometimes mildly decreased glucose levels. Elevations of ACE immunoglobulin G index, oligoclonal bands, CD4:CD8 lymphocyte ratios, and lysosyme and β2-microglobulin levels have been reported in CSF.[7] Approximately one-third of patients with neurosarcoidosis show normal CSF.[9,26-32] Moreover, in conditions, such as multiple sclerosis and systemic lupus erythematosus, similar CSF abnormalities may be found. CSF-ACE levels appear to be elevated in more than half of patients with neurosarcoidosis.[31,32]

In conclusion, determination of CSF-ACE level is not specific for neurosarcoidosis. High levels of CSF-ACE are not specific to neurosarcoidosis and have also been reported in CNS infections and malignant tumors. However, CSF-ACE level seems to be particularly useful in monitoring disease activity and response to treatment.

THERAPY OF NEUROSARCOIDOSIS

About two-thirds of patients with neurosarcoidosis have a self-limited monophasic illness; the rest have a chronic remitting-relapsing course. With treatment, death from neurologic disease is unusual. Although controlled studies are lacking, corticosteroids appear to reduce symptoms and size of granulomas, and it is unclear whether they affect the natural history.

The use of steroids depends on the clinical setting. Short-term therapy can be given to patients with aseptic meningitis or isolated facial palsy; long-term treatment is often necessary for intraparenchymal lesions, hydrocephalus, optic or other cranial nerve involvement, peripheral neuropathy, or symptomatic myopathy. Prednisone, 40–80 mg/day can be given for a few weeks and then slowly tapered either to a lowest possible maintenance dose or, if possible, to discontinuation. Higher initial doses may be necessary in some patients. Adjunctive immunosuppressive treatment for refractory patients includes azathioprine, methotrexate, cyclophosphamide, chlorambucil, and cyclosporine. Radiation therapy has been used with uncertain benefit.

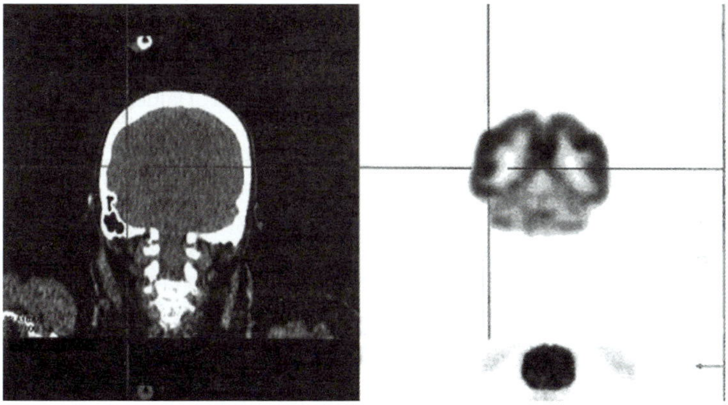

Figure 20-5 This is rare in sarcoidosis. 18 F-FDG PET is useful in finding other suitable sites for biopsy, and when the organ involvement has to be pursued. In a patient with chronic pulmonary and osseous sarcoidosis, frontal, occipital left, and temporal right accumulation of the FDG marker presenting lesions with active neurosarcoidosis. SUVmax = 4.3. The CSF-ACE level was 13 U/l. PET scan is not a method of choice in the diagnosis of neurosarcoidosis, however, in this patient the endocranial findings appeared unexpectedly. This is rare finding in sarcoidosis because the brain is not systematically included in whole body 18 F-FDG PET imaging. The main reason for this disadvantage of 18 F-FDG imaging in detecting central nervous system lesions is its high physiological uptake in the brain, which results in minimizing the lesion/brain ratio. The final result is that 18 F-FDG PET is considered to be of little interest in neurosarcoidosis and more often the brain is not included in the so-called "whole body" PET images. The suggestion is to include the brain in the PET scanning session. F-FDG, F-fluorodeoxyglucose; PET, positron emission tomography; SUVmax, maximum standardized uptake value per focus; CSF, cerebrospinal fluid; ACE, angiotensin converting enzyme. *Courtesy:* Professor Dragana Sobic-Saranovic, National PET Scan Center, Clinical Center Belgrade, Serbia.

REFERENCES

1. Delaney P. Neurologic manifestations in sarcoidosis: a review of literature with a report of 23 cases. *Ann Intern Med.* 1977;87:336-45.
2. James D, Sharma OP. Neurosarcoidosis. *Proc R Soc Med.* 1967;60:1169-73.
3. Mana J, Salazar A. Neurosarcoidosis: a report of 14 cases. *Sarcoidosis.* 1994;11:373.
4. Oksanen V. Neurosarcoidosis. In: James DG, editor. Sarcoidosis and other granulomatous disorders. New York: Marcel Dekker; 1994. Vol. 73. p. 285-309.
5. Scott T. Neurosarcoidosis: progress and clinical aspects. *Neurology.* 1993;43:8-12.
6. Sharma OP, Sharma A. Sarcoidosis of the nervous system. *Arch Intern Med.* 1991;151:1317-21.
7. Sharma OP. Neurosarcoidosis: a personal perspective based on a study of 38 patients. *Chest.* 1997;112:220-8.
8. Hoitsma E, Sharma OP. Neurosarcoidosis. In: Drent M, Costabel U, editors. European Respiratory Monograph: Sarcoidosis. European Respiratory Society; 2005. p. 164-87.
9. Mihailovic-Vucinic V, Sharma OP. Atlas of sarcoidosis pathogenesis, diagnosis and clinical features. London: Springer; 2005.
10. Hoitsma E, Marziniak M, Faber CG, Reulen JP, Sommer C, De Baets M, et al. Small fiber neuropathy in sarcoidosis. *Lancet.* 2002;359:2085-6.
11. Hoitsma E, Drent M, Verstraete E, Faber CG, Troost J, Spaans F, et al. Abnormal warm and cold sensation thresholds suggestive of small-fibre neuropathy in sarcoidosis. *Clin Neurophysiol.* 2003;114:2326-33.
12. Hoitsma E, Reulen JP, de Baets M, Drent M, Spaans F, Faber CG. Small fiber neuropathy: a common and important clinical disorder. *J Neurol Sci.* 2004;227:119-30.
13. Hoitsma E, Faber CG, van Kroonenburgh MJ, Gorgels AP, Halders SG, Heidendal GA, et al. Association of small fiber neuropathy with cardiac sympathetic dysfunction in sarcoidosis. *Sarcoidosis Vasc Diffuse Lung Dis.* 2005;22:43-50.
14. Polydefkis M, Allen RP, Hauer P, Earley CJ, Griffin JW, McArthur JC. Subclinical sensory neuropathy in late-onset restless legs syndrome. *Neurology.* 2000;55:1115-21.
15. Verbraecken J, Hoitsma E, van der Grinten CP, Cobben NA, Wouters EF, Drent M. Sleep disturbances associated with periodic leg movements in chronic sarcoidosis. *Sarcoidosis Vasc Diffuse Lung Dis.* 2004;21:137-46.
16. Hoitsma E, Faber CG, Drent M, Sharma OP. Neurosarcoidosis: a clinical dilemma. *Lancet Neurol.* 2004;3:397-407.
17. Sabaawi M, Gutierrez-Nunez J, Fragala MR. Neurosarcoidosis presenting as schizophreniform disorder. *Int J Psychiatry Med.* 1992;22:269-74.
18. Cahill DW, Salcman M. Neurosarcoidosis: a review of the rarer manifestations. *Surg Neurol.* 1981;15:204-11.
19. Cipri S, Gambardella G, Campolo C, Mannino R, Consoli D. Unusual clinical presentation of cerebral-isolated sarcoidosis. Case report and review of the literature. *J Neurosurg Sci.* 2000;44:140-4.
20. Jarman PR, Whyte MK, Glass DM, Peters AM. Case report: imaging of central nervous system sarcoidosis with gallium-67 single photon emission computed tomography. *Br J Radiol.* 1996;69:192-4.
21. Dubey N, Miletich RS, Wasay M, Mechtler LL, Bakshi R. Role of fluorodeoxyglucose positron emission tomography in the diagnosis of neurosarcoidosis. *J Neurol Sci.* 2002;205:77-81.
22. Davis LE, Kornfeld M. Neurocysticercosis: neurologic, pathogenetic, diagnostic and therapeutic aspects. *Eur Neurol.* 1991;31:229-40.

23. Nowak DA, Widenka DC. Neurosarcoidosis: a review of its intracranial manifestation. *J Neurol.* 2001;248:363-72.
24. Junger SS, Stern BJ, Levine SR, Sipos E, Marti-Masso JF. Intramedullary spinal sarcoidosis: clinical and magnetic resonance imaging characteristics. *Neurology.* 1993;43:333-7.
25. Kirmi O, Sheerin F, Patel N. Imaging of the meninges and the extra-axial spaces. *Semin Ultrasound CT MRI.* 2009;30:565-93.
26. McLean B, Miller D, Thompson E. Oligoclonal banding of IgG in CSF, blood-brain barrier function, and MRI findings in patients with sarcoidosis, systemic lupus erythematosus and Behcet disease involving the nervous system. *J Neurol Neurosurg Psychiatry.* 1995;58:548-54.
27. Scott TF, Seay AR, Goust JM. Pattern and concentration of IgG in cerebrospinal fluid in neurosarcoidosis. *Neurology.* 1989;39:1637-9.
28. Juozevicius JL, Rynes RI. Increased helper/suppressor T-lymphocyte ratio in the cerebrospinal fluid of a patient with neurosarcoidosis. *Ann Intern Med.* 1986;104:807-8.
29. Oksanen V, Gronhagen-Riska C, Tikanoja S, Somer H, Fyhrquist F. Cerebrospinal fluid lysozyme and b2-microglobulin in neurosarcoidosis. *J Neurol Sci.* 1986;73:79-87.
30. Tahmoush AJ, Amir MS, Connor WW, Farry JK, Didato S, Ulhoa-Cintra A, et al. CSF-ACE activity in probable CNS neurosarcoidosis. *Sarcoidosis Vasc Diffuse Lung Dis.* 2002;19:191-7.
31. Borucki SJ, Nguyen BV, Ladoulis CT, McKendall RR. Cerebrospinal fluid immunoglobulin abnormalities in neurosarcoidosis. *Arch Neurol.* 1989;46:270-3.
32. Lynch JP 3rd. Neurosarcoidosis: how good are the diagnostic tests? *J Neuroophthalmol.* 2003;23:187-9.

CHAPTER

21 Headache in Sarcoidosis

INTRODUCTION

Although clinical manifestations of neurosarcoidosis can be vague, headaches are frequently reported in neurosarcoidosis (30%).[1,2]

The data from the literature, however, vary depending on the emphasis the authors give to this symptom and evidence-based data suggest this symptom might be more common than previously realized (72–92%).[3,4]

HISTORICAL ACCOUNT

The first and probably the most notable description of nervous system involvement in sarcoidosis was reported by Danish ophthalmologist Frederic Heerfordt in 1909, in a description of patients with uveitis, parotid gland enlargement, and facial nerve palsies during the course of febrile condition. Presently, the condition is named "febris uveoparotidea subchronica" or "Heerfordt's syndrome".[5]

CLINICAL MANIFESTATIONS OF HEADACHE IN SARCOIDOSIS

A headache defined as a pain in the head or upper neck and is one of the most common locations of pain in the body. Headache has many causes. According to the International Classification of Headache Disorders 2nd edition, headaches are classified into three major categories:

1. Primary headaches: tension headaches—the most common; migraine headaches—second most common type; and cluster headaches—rare type of primary headache.
2. Secondary headache: due to underlying problem within the head and neck.
3. Cranial neuralgias, facial pain, and others[6]

SECONDARY HEADACHE

The subcommittee of the International Headache Society for headache classification (ICHD-II) has recently recognized that secondary headaches may occur in patients affected by inflammatory disease of the central nervous system (CNS). These headaches are classified into 4 main groups depending on the disease in which they occur:[6]

- Neurosarcoidosis
- Aseptic (noninfectious) meningitis
- Other noninfectious inflammatory diseases
- Lymphocytic hypophysitis.

The incidence of nervous system involvement in general population of sarcoidosis patients is estimated to be approximately 5–15%.[7]

Evidence of neurosarcoidosis is particularly difficult because in the majority of patients, neurological symptoms are frequently the first manifestations of the disease.[8,9] Headache might be the prominent symptom. The following lesions of nervous system might cause headaches in patients with sarcoidosis.

Lesions of Neurosarcoidosis Causing Secondary Headaches

Dura Based Lesions Causing Headache in Sarcoidosis

Differential diagnosis in patients presenting with dural thickening should include other causes of chronic meningitis as presented in table 21-1.

Leptomeningeal Involvement

Occasionally, it may present with headache as a prominent symptom. As leptomeningeal infiltrations are usually found at suprasellar and frontal basal meninges or sometimes at the region of chiasm, or floor of the third ventricle, clinical symptoms usually correlate with these locations on the magnetic resonance imaging (Figure 21-1). The differential diagnosis of headache in sarcoidosis caused by leptomeningeal involvement is given in table 21-2.

Enhancing Brain Parenchymal Lesions Causing Headaches in Sarcoidosis

Besides seizures,[11] the most common symptom occurring with enhancing brain parenchymal lesion in recurrent headache, although these patients can also experience diabetes insipidus or hypopituitarismus.

Granulomas in the subependymal layers of the ventricular system are possible cause of hydrocephalus in neurosarcoidosis (Figure 21-2).[10,12] Intraparenchymal granulomas that are usually associated with small blood vessels (veins or/and arteries) suggest that granulomatous lesions of sarcoidosis infiltrate brain through vascular

Table 21-1 Differential Diagnosis of Headache in Sarcoidosis due to Dural Thickening[10]
Meningeoma
Lymphoma
Adenocarcinoma
Wegener's idiopathic hypertrophic cranial pachymeningitis
Granulomatous infections
Leukemia

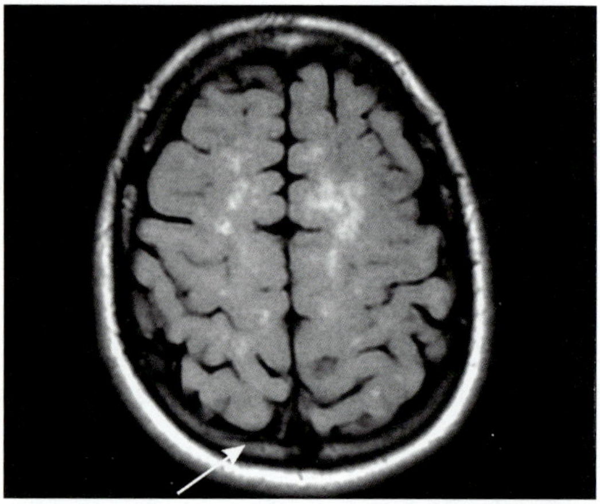

Figure 21-1 Meningeal involvement in sarcoidosis (arrows). Besides meningeal thickening the magnetic resonance imaging revealed diffuse parenchymal lesions. This patient suffered for years from headache as the dominant symptom of her sarcoidosis.

Table 21-2 Differential Diagnosis of Headache in Sarcoidosis Caused by Leptomeningeal Involvement[10]
Tuberculosis
Wegener's granulomatous meningitis
Fungal meningitis
Pyogenic meningitis
Leptomeningeal lymphoma
Dermyelination
Meningoangiomatosis
Acute lymphocytic leukemia
Leptomeningeal carcinomatosis

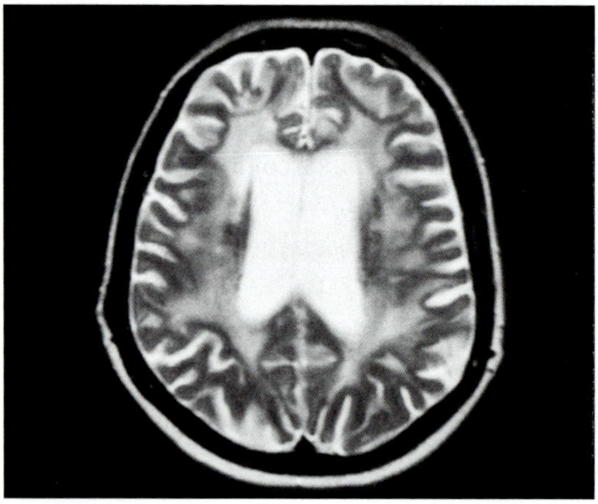

Figure 21-2: Hydrocephalus in sarcoidosis. Very rare but possible cause of headache.

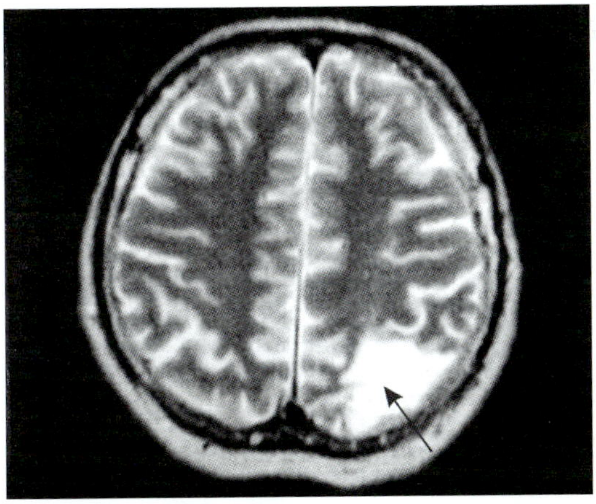

Figure 21-3 A 43-year-old patient with chronic pulmonary sarcoidosis and chronic headache. Magnetic resonance imaging contrast-enhanced T1-weighted image showed left parietal mass (arrow). Noncaseating granulomas were seen at biopsy. The patient's symptoms resolved with steroids.

spaces.[10] It is thus quite difficult to distinguish sarcoid angiitis from primary angiitis of CNS) in a biopsy tissue.[10,13] Sarcoidosis patients with enhancing brain parenchymal lesions often have recurrence of symptoms, or the symptoms do not change under therapy, so chronic lasting headache may occur (Figure 21-3). Although prednisolone usually lessens the headache, 75% of these patients are resistant to treatment.[10]

Nonenhancing Brain Parenchymal Lesions

Granulomatous angiopathy may cause small areas of infarction located as nonspecific periventricular lesions. The lesions may also occur in multiple sclerosis, hypertension, and vasculitis. Headache may be a prominent symptom in patients with granulomatous angiopathy as well as in patients with hypertension and/or vasculitis.[10] Diffuse cerebral vasculopathy can cause stroke-like episodes with headache as prominent symptom.[7,14]

CRANIAL NEURALGIAS AND FACIAL PAIN IN SARCOIDOSIS

Facial pain can be the presenting and sometimes even the only complaint in sarcoidosis. Differential diagnosis of facial pain can be difficult.

An approach based on history and neurologic examination allows working diagnosis to be made at the bed side. Facial pain with cranial nerves involvement requires urgent examination.

PAINFUL OPHTHALMOPLEGIA

Sarcoid inflammation of the eye (iridicyclitis and uveitis) is often accompanied by severe, unilateral pain in the eye or around it. The pain is usually associated with red eye and papillary abnormalities.

Table 21-3 Possible Inflammatory Causes of Painful Ophatalmoplegia[15]
Ocular myositis
Idiopathic inflammatory pseudotumor of the orbit
Tolosa-Hunt syndrome
Wegener's granulomatosis
Systemic lupus erythematosus
Rheumatoid arthritis

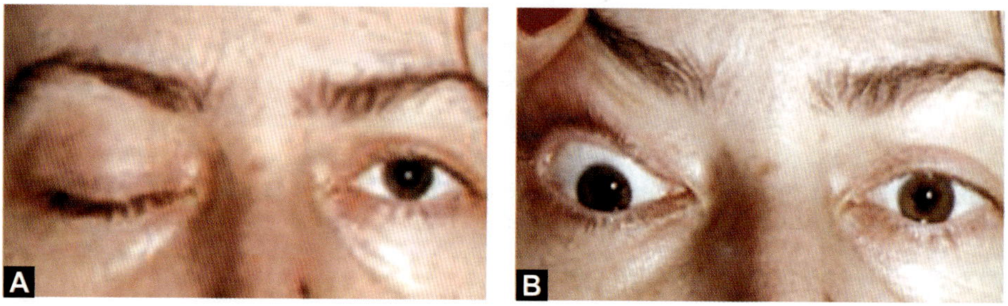

Figure 21-4 Patient with ocular motor palsy. Besides this manifestation, the patient experienced migraine like headache episodes.

Rarely, the modality seen in sarcoidosis is "ophthalmoplegic migraine" that includes migraine-like headache of long-duration and ocular motor palsy (Table 21-3 and Figure 21-4).[15]

REFERENCES

1. La Mantia L, Erbetta A. Headache and inflammatory disorders of the central nervous system. *Neurol Sci.* 2004;25:148-53.
2. Sharma O. Neurosarcoidosis: a personal perspective based on the study of 37 patients. *Chest.* 1997;112;220-8.
3. Zajicek JP, Scolding NJ, Foster O, Rovaris M, Evanson J, Mooseley IF, et al. Central nervous system sarcoidosis--diagnosis and management. *QJM.* 1999;92:103-17.
4. Vucinic-Mihailovic V, Rasulic L, Stjepanovic M, Filipovic S. Neurosarcoidosis: MRI and CSF findings in our patients. Abstracts of the WASOGBAL 2011 conference. Abstract C7.
5. Sharma O. Sarcoidosis: a historical perspective. *Clin Dermatol.* 2007;25:232-41.
6. The International Classification of Headache Disorders, 2nd Edition (ICHD-II)--revision of criteria for 8.2 Medication-overuse headache. *Cephalalgia.* 2005;25:460-5.
7. Hoitsma E, Drent M, Sharma OP. A pragmatic approach to diagnosing and treating neurosarcoidosis in the 21st century. *Curr Opin Pulm Med.* 2010;16:472-9.
8. Joseph FG, Scolding NJ. Neurosarcoidosis: a study of 30 new cases. *J Neurol Neurosurg Psychiatry.* 2009;80:297-304.
9. Shah R, Robertson GH, Cure JK. Correlation of MR imaging findings and clinical manifestations in neurosarcoidosis. *Am J Neuroradiol.* 2009;30:953-61.
10. Christoforidis G, Spickler E, Recio M, Mehta B. MR of CNS sarcoidosis: correlation of imaging. features to clinical symptoms and response to treatment. *AJNR Am J Neuroradiol.* 1999;20:655-69.

11. Krumholz A, Stern BJ, Stern EG. Clinical implications of seizures in neurosarcoidosis. *Arch Neurol.* 1991;48:842-4.
12. Lexa FJ, Grossman RI. MR of sarcoidosis in the head and spine: spectrum of manifestations and radiographic response to steroid therapy. *AJNR Am J Neuroradiol.* 1994;15:973-82
13. Lee SC, Spencer J, Rumberg J, Dickson DW. Isolated central nervous system granulomatosis resembling sarcoidosis. *Neurology.* 1989;236:356-8.
14. Brisman JL, Hinduja A, McKinney JS, Gerhardstein B. Successful urgent angioplasty of neruosarcoid vasculitis presenting with strokes. *Surg Neurol.* 2006;66:402-4.
15. Siccoli MM, Bassetti C, Sándor P. Facial pain: clinical differential diagnosis. *Lancet Neurol.* 2006;5:257-67.

CHAPTER

22 Hematological Changes in Sarcoidosis

Various mechanisms cause the hematological changes seen in sarcoidosis.[1-4]

- Granulomatous involvement of the bone marrow
- Sequestration of blood cells in the spleen
- Immunologic destruction of the peripheral blood elements.

Peripheral eosinophilia is commonly found in sarcoidosis. Five to thirty-five percent of the patients may have eosinophillia greater than 5% and the absolute percentage in any patients can be as high as 67%. No proven or postulated mechanism has been described as yet for this eosinophilia.[1-6]

Leukopenia (white blood cell count less than 3,000/mm^3) is quite common in sarcoidosis (28–41%).[1-6]

Lymphopenia is also common with the significantly lower total counts and higher suppressor cell ($CD8^+$) percentages. Rarely, a profound lymphopenia raises a concern of HIV disease.[7]

Thrombocytopenia is the least common abnormality in sarcoidosis (1.3%), and is probably due to immune mediated mechanisms-platelet associated antibodies and sequestration in patients with splenomegaly and pancytopenia.[1-6] Sarcoidosis associated with idiopathic thrombocytopenic purpura (ITP) or autoimmune hemolytic anemia is rare.[8] One report documented the usefulness of high dose steroids to treat ITP associated with sarcoidosis.[9]

Pancytopenia may be caused by hypersplenism, or bone marrow infiltration with granulomas (Figure 22-1).

Raised serum angiotensin converting enzyme level is a good test to monitor course of the disease and response to treatment (Figure 22-2). Serum angiotensin converting enzyme (ACE) determination is the most widely used biochemical test in sarcoidosis. The test has a low sensitivity, because increased levels are found only in about 60% of sarcoidosis patients. Changes in serum ACE levels reflect the course of the granulomatous process. Resolution of the active disease or clinical control of sarcoidosis by adequate corticosteroid therapy brings serum ACE level down to the normal range.

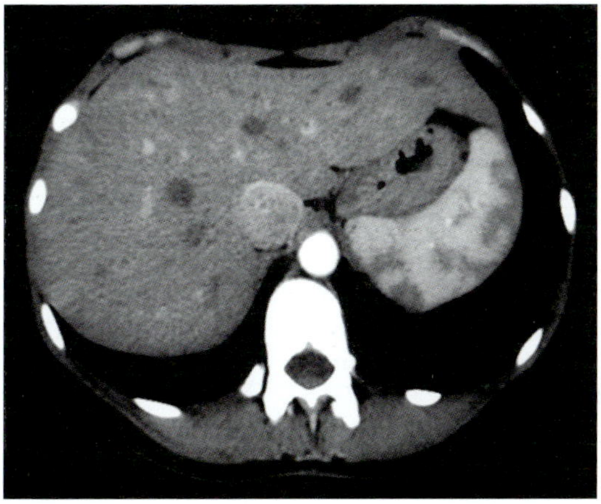

Figure 21-1 Liver and spleen involvement in sarcoidosis patient with pancytopenia. Patient also had bone marrow granulomas.

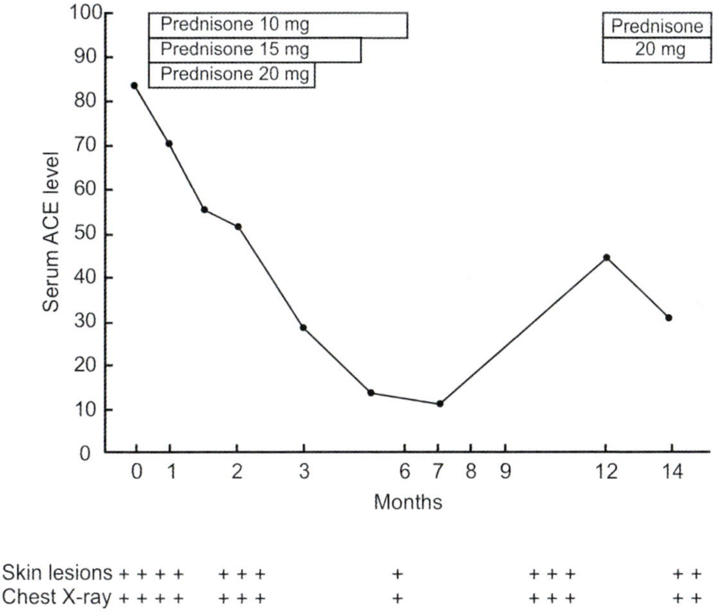

Figure 22-2 The serum angiotensin converting enzyme determinations are useful for monitoring the course of the disease and respond to treatment. ACE, angiotensin converting enzymes. *Source* Sharma OP. Sarcoidosis: Clinical Management. London: Butterworths; 1984, p. 151

REFERENCES

1. Lower EE, Smith JT, Martelo OJ, Baughman RP. The anemia of sarcoidosis. *Sarcoidosis.* 1988;5:51-5.
2. Kennedy D, Yamakido M. Hematologic manifestations of sarcoidosis. *Semin Resp Med.* 1992;13:455-8.

3. Means R Jr. Pathogenesis of the anemia of chronic disease; a cytokine-mediated anemia. *Stem Cell.* 1995;13:32-7.
4. Browne P, Sharma O, Salkin D. Bone marrow sarcoidosis. *JAMA.* 1978;240:43-50.
5. Dieckerman J, Holbrook P, Zinkman W. Etiology and therapy of thrombocytopenia associated with sarcoidosis. *J Pediatr.* 1972;81:758-64.
6. Lawrence H, Greenberg B. Autoimmune thrombocytopenia in sarcoidosis. *Am J Med.* 1985;79:761-4.
7. Lenner R, Bregman Z, Teirstein AS, DePalo L. Recurrent pulmonary sarcoidosis in HIV-infected patients receiving highly active antiretroviral therapy. *Chest.* 2001;119:978-81.
8. Kondo H, Sakai S, Sakai Y. Autoimmune haemolytic anaemia, Sjogren's syndrome and idiopathic thrombocytopenic purpura in a patient with sarcoidosis. *Acta Haematol* 1993;89:209-12.
9. Chakrabarti S, Behera D, Varma S, Bambery P. High-dose methyl prednisolone for autoimmune thrombocytopenia in sarcoidosis. *Sarcoidosis Vasc Diffuse Lung Dis.* 1997;14:188.

CHAPTER

23 Bone and Bone Marrow Involvement

INTRODUCTION

Lung involvement is frequently reported in sarcoidosis and more than 90% of patients have combination of lung, skin, or eye involvement.

However, osseous lesions are less commonly reported in sarcoidosis, but when present, bone affection usually signifies chronic persistent and progressive disease.

BONE

Frequency of bone involvement varies between 3–13% and usually has bilateral distribution. The site of bone involvement is cortical with the periosteum remaining preserved and with the most commonly affected bones being hands and feet. The bony lesions are typically cystic with minimal disturbance of surrounding soft tissue, and usually can be easily appreciated on radiographic imaging (Figure 23-1). The lesions typically involve the middle and proximal phalanges with usual sparing of the metacarpal bones. Other lesions include permeative lesions that lead to "tunneling" of the cortex with subsequent remodeling, transforming the concave structure into a tubular one. These lesions are usually accompanied by soft tissue swelling and

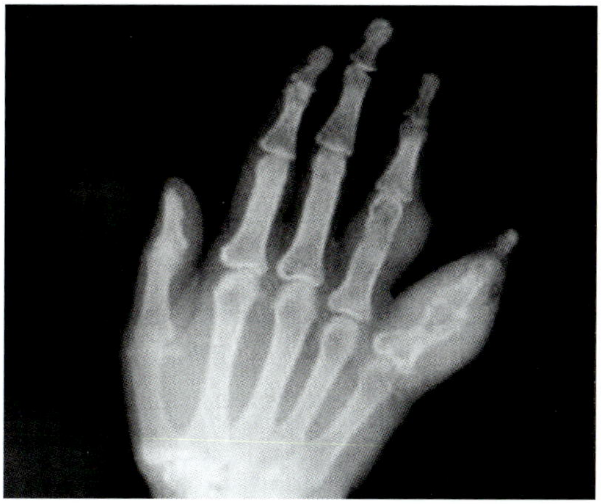

Figure 23-1 Bone cysts and destruction accompanied by soft tissue swelling in sarcoidosis.

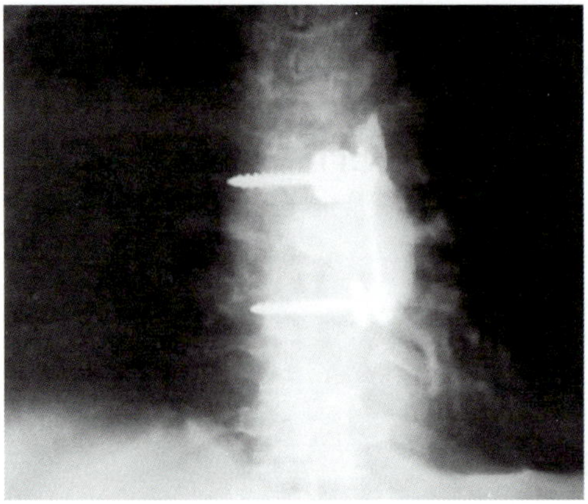

Figure 23-2 Patients may have vertebral sarcoidosis, a rare locations. A needle or open biopsy is indicated to make the diagnosis. The metal graft represented in this patient is used to stabilize the vertebral bones.

have a propensity for fractures. Nasal bones may be involved in patients with lupus pernio. Involvement of the skull, sternum, ribs, pelvis, and distal ends of long bones is rare. Rarely, patients may have vertebral sarcoidosis, in which case, a needle or open biopsy is indicated to make the diagnosis (Figure 23-2). The imaging studies in these patients may show sclerotic lesions often indistinguishable from metastatic disease.

BONE MARROW GRANULOMAS: A SILENT PRESENTATION OF SARCOIDOSIS

Bone marrow granuloma is a common laboratory finding. The incidence ranges from 0.3–2.2% depending on the composition and origin of the series.[1] A review of 58 cases of bone marrow granuloma at a single institution over a 20-year period concluded that bone marrow granulomas were not only infrequently recognized but the pathologic finding also required extensive evaluation to find an underlying etiology.[2]

There are many illnesses that cause marrow granulomas. In a multisystem disease, bone granulomas are similar to the granulomas involving other organs. There are no reliable morphologic features that allow differentiation between the causes of bone marrow granuloma. Nevertheless, mycobacterial infections are usually the primary consideration. By combining histologic, microbiologic, and serologic techniques, an etiology can be documented in 90% of the patients.

Certain specific pathologic findings, however, are important, e.g., caseation in tuberculosis, necrosis with eosinophils in fungal diseases and vasculitis, Reed-Steinberg cells in Hodgkin's lymphoma, poorly organized granulomas in brucellosis and human immunodeficiency virus (HIV) infections, and "donut" granulomas in

Q-fever. If the diagnosis cannot be established on the histological appearance, an epidemiologic, occupational, and the drug-use and abuse-history usually provide a missing clue. Foreign bodies can be present in the bone marrow granulomas.

Silicosis and coal workers' pneumoconiosis have been reported in association with bone marrow granuloma. In coal workers, a characteristic yellow-brown pigment is found in the granuloma. The most commonly implicated drugs are procainamide and amiodarone. About 10% of the cases of bone marrow granuloma are of undetermined origin. Many of these cases most likely represent sarcoidosis without lung involvement. Steroid therapy improves the outcome in such patients[3,4] (Table 23-1).

Table 23-1 Important Causes of Bone Marrow Granulomas
Infectious diseases
Bacterial (tuberculosis, brucellosis, and Q-fever)
Fungal (histoplasmosis, coccidioidomycosis, and cryptococcosis)
Viral (cytomegalovirus and Epstein–Barr virus)
Malignant diseases
Lymphoma (Hodgkin's and non-Hodgkin's) disease
Metastatic carcinoma (colon, lung breast, sarcoma, and leukemia)
Drugs
Procainamide
Chlorpropamide
Allopurinol
Phenytoin
Amiodarone
Sulfonamides
Autoimmune
Rheumatoid arthritis
Systemic lupus erythematosus
Foreign bodies
Silicosis
Coal-worker's pneumoconiosis
Berylliosis
Intravenous drug abuse
Miscellaneous
Sarcoidosis
Behcet's disease
Familial Mediterranean fever
Idiopathic diffuse granulomatosis

Initial tests should include purified-protein derivative skin test, a direct acid fast bacilli (AFB) stain sputum (if applicable), bone marrow cultures for AFB and brucella organisms, cultures for various fungi, and a chest computed tomography (CT)/high resolution CT (HRCT) film. In addition, serologic tests should be done for *H. capsulatum* and *Coccidioides immitis* in endemic areas for these fungi. Serologic testing for HIV is indicated if the diagnosis of disseminated tuberculosis, histoplasmosis, or *M. avium* intracellulare is made or if the patient belongs to a high-risk group. The search for lymphoma including immunophenotyping of the bone marrow should be carried out. A search for brucellosis, typhoid fever, and Q fever should depend on clinical findings, origin of the patient, and travel history.[5]

A high angiotensin converting enzyme level, although nonspecific, supports the diagnosis of sarcoidosis. Corticosteroids reverse anemia and leucopenia noted in these patients. Fevers, chills, and joint pains subside. In addition, repeated bone marrow examination may also show substantial decrease in the number of granulomas and hyalinization of many of the remaining ones.[6]

The presence of noncaseating granulomas on the bone marrow examination should alert the physician to the possibility of sarcoidosis. Although the lungs are involved in 90–95% of sarcoidosis cases the presence of a normal chest roentgenogram should not make a clinician overlook the diagnosis of sarcoidosis.[7]

CASE STUDY

A 46-year-old woman came to a physician's office for diagnosis and management of a diffuse maculopapular rash and arthritis of her wrists and joints. Chest X-ray film was normal, but X-ray films of the hands showed "punched" bone cysts. Liver and bone marrow biopsies showed noncaseating granulomas (Figure 23-3). The long-term follow-up stretching over 30 years showed persistent anemia, leucopenia, and relative lymphocytosis (Figure 23-4). The patient died of natural death at the age of 86 years.

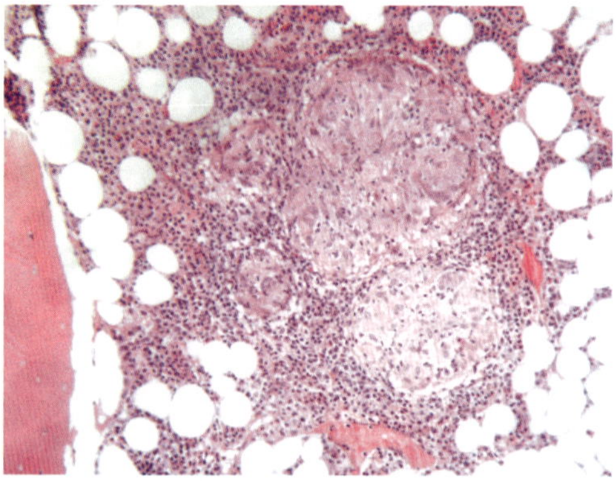

Figure 23-3 Bone marrow granuloma in patient with sarcoidosis.

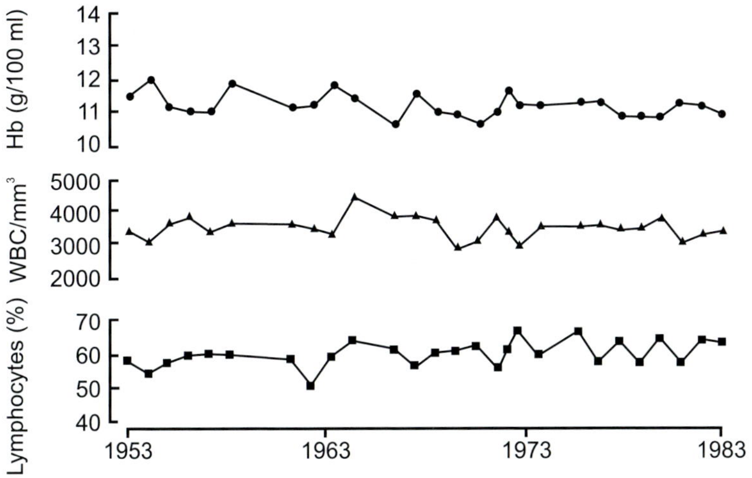

Figure 23-4 Leucopenia in a sarcoidosis patient lasting for more than 20 years. The patient had no symptoms or infections.Hb, hemoglobin; WBC, white blood cell. *Source:* Sharma OP. Sarcoidosis: Clinical Management. London: Butterworths; 1984. p. 87.

REFERENCES

1. Gormsen H. The occurrence of epithelioid cell granulomas in human bone marrow. *Acta Med Scand.* 1948;131:154-64.
2. Bodem CR, Hamory BH, Taylor HM, Kleopfer L. Granulomatous bone marrow disease. A review of the literature and clinicopathologic analysis of 58 cases. *Medicine (Baltimore).* 1983;62:372-83.
3. Eid A, Carion W, Nystrom JS. Differential diagnose of bone marrow granuloma. *West J Med.* 1996;164:510-5.
4. Kadin ME, Donaldson SS, Dorfman RF. Isolated granulomas in Hodgkin's disease. *N Engl J Med.* 1970;283:859-61.
5. Longcope WT, Freiman DG. A study of sarcoidosis; based on a combined investigation of 160 cases including 30 autopsies from The Johns Hopkins Hospital and Massachusetts General Hospital. *Medicine (Baltimore).* 1952;31:1-132.
6. Proceedings of the international conference on sarcoidosis. *Am Rev Respir Dis.* 1961; 84:1-183.
7. Brown P, Sharma O, Salkin D. Bone marrow sarcoidosis. *JAMA.* 1978;240:2654-5.

CHAPTER

24 Calcium Metabolism Disorders in Sarcoidosis

INTRODUCTION

Hypercalcemia is an important complication of sarcoidosis resulting from overproduction of 1, 25-dihydroxyvitamin D_3 [1,25$(OH)_2D_3$] (calcitriol) by activated macrophages and sarcoidosis granulomas. Calcitriol in turn causes increased absorption of calcium from the gut. Hypercalcemia is not specific to sarcoidosis for it is also found in other granulomatous disorders, including tuberculosis, coccidioidomycosis, histoplasmosis, leprosy, and granulomatous necrotizing vasculitis.

The kidneys may be affected primarily by sarcoid granulomas or secondarily from hypercalcemia, hypercalciuria, and nephrocalcinosis. Hypercalcemia and hypercalciuria appear to be important clinical features of sarcoidosis resulting from overproduction of calcitriol by activated macrophages and sarcoidosis granulomas.[1]

Calcium homeostasis is primarily controlled by levels of vitamin D, parathyroid hormone, and calcitonin; moreover it is also influenced by thyroid gland and sexual hormones. In sarcoidosis, there is deregulation of these mechanisms, leading to clinically manifested problems.

DISORDERS OF CALCIUM METABOLISM IN SARCOIDOSIS

Hypercalcemia and hypercalciuria are the most frequently observed disorders of calcium metabolism in sarcoidosis.

Hypercalcemia

Hypercalcemia is one of the most common biochemical abnormalities found in clinical practice. Serum hypercalcemia may be discovered when the serum calcium level is measured as a screening test or as a part of the evaluation for fatigue, unexplained weakness, neuromuscular disability, renal stones, or osteopenia.

The three most common causes of hypercalcemia are:

1. Hyperparathyroidism
2. Malignancy
3. Vitamin D mediated conditions.

Less common causes include milk alkali syndrome, immobilization, Addison disease, vitamin A intoxication, other granulomatous diseases, primary or secondary hyperthyroidism, Paget's disease, parenteral nutrition, and drug induced (thiazide, lithium, theophylline, and aspirine).[2]

Although hypercalcemia appears to be a feature of sarcoidosis, studies showing an excessively high frequency of occurrence need to be revised. It is reasonably to accept the incidence of 11% noted by James et al. in their worldwide review of 3,676 patients with sarcoidosis.[3]

Hypercalcemia is usually transient in subacute sarcoidosis and persistent and fluctuating in chronic disease, depending on the activity of the disease. Hypercalcemia may occur only at a certain phase during the long course of chronic sarcoidosis.[4]

There is no evidence that race, age, sex, occupation, or geographic distribution influences the development of hypercalcemia.[3]

Long-standing hypercalcemia and hypercalciuria in sarcoidosis can cause nephrocalcinosis and nephrolithiasis which occurs in over half the patients with sarcoidosis who have renal impairment and is the major cause of chronic renal failure.[5]

Symptoms and signs of hypercalcemia are related to the degree of elevation of the serum calcium concentration, the rapidity of its development, and its cause. Mild hypercalcemia (serum calcium 10–11.5 mg/dL) is usually asymptomatic and well tolerated. Moderate hypercalcemia (11.5–13.5 mg/dL) and severe hypercalcemia (more than 13.5 mg/dL, also called hypercalcemia crisis) are associated with progressive symptoms of fatigue, polyuria, weakness, anorexia, nausea, vomiting, constipation, abdominal pain, change in mental status, lethargy, and, if left untreated, coma. Electrocardiographic changes, such as QT interval shortening and arrhythmias are common in patients with severe hypercalcemia. There is a report of ST-segment elevations in electrocardiogram in patients with severe hypercalcemia.[5]

Calcium levels greater than 14–15 mg/dL can cause life-threatening cardiac arrhythmias.[2]

Hypercalciuria

Although hypercalcemia has long been recognized as a complication of sarcoidosis, the importance of hypercalciuria has been less thoroughly realized. However, hypercalciuria is 3 times more common than hypercalcemia. Sharma et al. reported that the possible incidence of hypercalcemia in sarcoidosis ranges from 2 to 63%.[4,6,7]

Hypercalciuria has been reported to be more common in males than in females. Three different mechanisms are responsible for hypercalciuria:

1. Absorptive: this type of hypercalcemia is associated with elevated calcitriol levels and abnormal urinary calcium: creatinine ratio.
2. Resorptive: associated with excessive dissemination of sarcoidosis involving bones; this type of hypercalcemia is associated with high serum angiotensin converting enzyme levels.
3. Associated with osteoclasts activating factor (bone resolving substance).[1]

Persistent hypercalciuria may lead to nephrocalcinosis, renal stones, obstruction of the collecting tubules, and finally renal failure. Rizzato referred 36% out of his patients with renal stones as presenting features of sarcoidosis.[8] Persistent hypercalciuria may lead to nephrocalcinosis, renal stones, obstruction of the collecting tubules, and finally renal failure (Figure 24-1).

Hamada and colleagues found renal impairments predominantly in patients with hypercalcemia; nephocalcinosis was not present in all cases.[9]

MANAGEMENT OF CALCIUM METABOLISM IMPAIRMENTS IN SARCOIDOSIS

Corticosteroid therapy is an effective in treatment of hypercalcemia (Figure 24-2),[12,13] because corticosteroids may exacerbate hypercalciuria at the very beginning of the treatment, the suggestion is to control urinary calcium excretion after beginning of therapy (Figure 24-3). It is accepted that corrected serum calcium concentration of >3.0 mmoL/L or evidence of renal complications is an indication for therapy. Patients with uncomplicated hypercalcemia of <3.0 mmoL/L probably do not require immediate treatment but should be followed up carefully because calcium levels fluctuate.[10]

The early management of severe hypercalcemia involves rehydration to correct volume depletion, a loop diuretic to encourage renal calcium secretion, and corticosteroids because of their effectiveness in rapidly restoring normocalcemia.

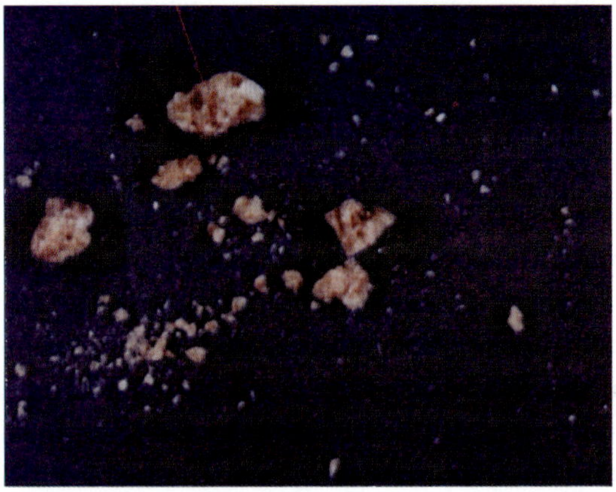

Figure 24-1 The stones passed in the urine of a sarcoidosis patient with hypercalciuria.

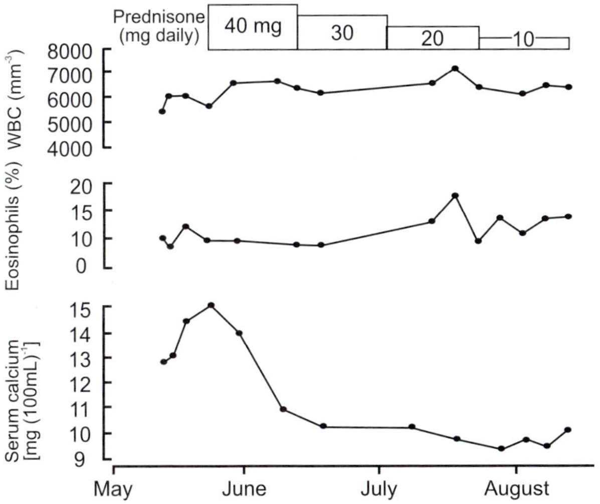

Figure 24-2 Hypercalcemia is present in about 13% of sarcoidosis patients. Hypercalcemia responded to prednisone therapy, however, in this patient, peripheral eosinophillia persisted. WBC, white blood cell. *Source:* Sharma OP. Sarcoidosis: Clinical Management. London: Butterworths; 1984. p. 82.

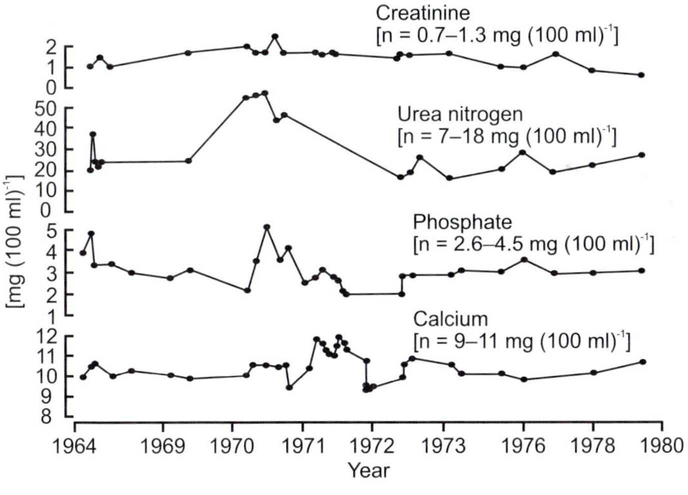

Figure 24-3 Serum calcium and renal function in sarcoidosis patient with chronic, persistent disease. Follow-up for more than 16 years, notice that hypercalcemia occurred only during one phase of the disease and would have been easily missed had the serum calcium levels not been so carefully monitored. *Source:* Sharma OP. Sarcoidosis: Clinical Management. London: Butterworths; 1984. p. 148.

Although corticosteroids have no effect on 1-α hydroxylase in the renal tubular cell, they are inhibitors of this enzyme in the macrophages.[11]

They normalize by down regulating interleukin-2 and interferon-γ expression. In practice, patients with hypercalcemia are advised to minimize their exposure to sunlight, avoid vitamin D rich food, and maintain a fluid intake of more than 2 L/day.

Corticosteroid therapy is an effective in treatment of hypercalcemia,[12,13] because corticosteroids may exacerbate hypercalciuria at the very beginning of the treatment; the suggestion is to control urinary calcium excretion after beginning of therapy. Patients in whom corticosteroids are contraindicated may be treated with ketoconasole. Ketoconazole has been used in primarily hyperparathyroidism in order to reduce calcitriol synthesis.[14]

However, the use of ketoconazole in combination with corticosteroids for treating hypercalcemia in sarcoidosis patients is limited to isolated case reports.[15]

Hydroxychloroquine also causes inhibition of 25(OH)3-1-α hydroxylase and can be considered in treating patients who cannot tolerate ketoconazole or patients with side effects of it (i.e., impaired liver function).[16]

Methotrexate and azathioprine are frequently used in the treatment of sarcoidosis. They do not have any particular effect on calcium metabolism, but they can help the control of hypercalcemia by reducing the total granuloma burden.

OSTEOPOROSIS IN SARCOIDOSIS PATIENTS

The primary or/and secondary prevention of glucocorticoid-induced osteoporosis is quite difficult in patients with sarcoidosis because of the coexisting impairments of calcium and vitamin D metabolism, as illustrated most recently in an outstanding review of Sweiss et al.[17]

This is the study on bone health problems in sarcoidosis, with the emphasis of vitamin D metabolism disorders. Besides elucidating the problem of calcium metabolism and the vitamin D disorders in sarcoidosis, authors highlighted the problem of treatment of steroid induced osteoporosis giving the accurate, evidence-based suggestions.

However, because of potential hypercalciuria and hypercalcemia, the usual conservative treatment for low bone mass, calcium and vitamin D supplements, may not be well tolerated. No prediction model is adequate. Each patient needs to be assessed individually, including measurement of body mass index, serum and urine calcium, and sex steroid status.[17]

REFERENCES

1. Sharma OP. Renal sarcoidosis and hypercalcaemia. *Eur Respir Mon.* 2005;32:220-32.
2. Desai HV, Gandhi K, Sharma M, Jennine M, Singh P, Brogan M. Thiazide-induced severe hypercalcemia: a case report and review of literature. *Am J Ther.* 2010;17:e234-6.
3. James DG, Neville E, Siltzbach L. A worldwide view of sarcoidosis. *Ann N Y Acad Sci.* 1976;278:321-34.
4. Sharma O, Trowell J, Cohen N, et al. Abnormal calcium metabolism in sarcoidosis. In: Turiaf J, Chabot J, editors. La Sarcoidose: Rapports de IV Conference Internationale

(Proceedings of the IV International Conference on Sarcoidosis). Paris: Maison et Cie; 1967. p. 627-31.
5. Monge M, Miquel O, Dugardin F, Modeliar SS, Glérant JC, Hacène S, et al. Sarcoidosis and the kidney: not only the granulomatous interstitial nephritis. *Clin Nephrol.* 2009;71:192-5.
6. Sharma O. Hypercalcemia in granulomatous disorders: a clinical review. *Curr Opin Pulm Med.* 2000;6:442-7.
7. Sharma OP. Vitamin D, calcium, and sarcoidosis. *Chest.* 1996;109:535-9.
8. Rizzato G, Palmieri G, Agrati A, Zanussi C. The organ-specific extrapulmonary presentation of sarcoidosis: a frequent occurrence but a challenge to an early diagnosis. A 3-year-long prospective observational study. *Sarcoidosis Vasc Diffuse Lung Dis.* 2004;21:119-26.
9. Hamada H, Nagai S, Ono T, Muso E, Nagao T, Shigematsu M, et al. Sarcoidosis complicated with IgA nephropathy. *Sarcoidosis Vasc Diffuse Lung Dis.* 2003;20:69-73.
10. Conron M, Young C, Beyon H. Calcium metabolism in sarcoidosis and its clinical implications. *Rheumatology (Oxford).* 2000;39:707-13
11. Adamas J Gacad M. Characterisation of 1 alfa hydroxylation of vitamin D sterols by cultured alveolar macrophages from patients with sarcoidosis. *J Exp Med.* 1985;161:755-65.
12. Rizzato G. Clinical impact of bone and calcium metabolism changes in sarcoidosis. *Thorax.* 1998;53:425–9.
13. Rizzato, G. Calcium metabolism. In: Baughman R, editor. Sarcoidosis. New York: Taylor & Francis; 2006. p. 635-51.
14. Glass AR, Eil C. Ketoconasole induced reduction in serum 1,25 dihydroxyvitamin D and total serum calcium in hypercalcemic patients. *J Clin Endocrinol Metab.* 1988;66:934-8.
15. Adams J, Sharma OP, Diz MM, Endres DB. Ketoconasole decreases the serum 1,25 dihydroxyvitamin D and calcium concentration in sarcoidosis-associated hypercalcemia. *J Clin Endocrinol Metab.* 1990;70:1090-5.
16. O'Leary TJ, Jones G, Yip A, Lohnes D, Cohanim M, Yendt ER. The effects of chloroquine on serum 1,25 dihydroxyvitamin D and calcium metabolism in sarcoidosis. *Engl J Med.* 1986;315:727-30.
17. Sweiss NJ, Lower EE, Korsten P, Niewold TB, Favus MJ, Baughman RP. Bone health issues in sarcoidosis. *Curr Rheumatol Rep.* 2011;13:265-72.

CHAPTER

25 Renal Sarcoidosis

INTRODUCTION

The kidneys are less frequently affected by sarcoidosis than other organs. Nevertheless, physicians taking care of sarcoidosis patients need to be aware of the possibility of renal involvement in order to diagnose this potentially fatal complication early and treat it effectively. The kidneys may be affected primarily by sarcoid granulomas or secondarily from hypercalcemia, hypercalciuria, and nephrocalcinosis.

INCIDENCE

Clinically manifest renal involvement is rare in sarcoidosis.[1-4] The reported prevalence of renal disease ranges widely due to the enormous variation in study designs and enrolled patient populations (Table 25-1).

Several small series of biopsy findings suggest that some degree of renal involvement occurs in approximately 35–50% of patients with chronic sarcoidosis, but rarely in those with acute sarcoidosis.[4-7]

Table 25-1 Organ Involvement (%) in Sarcoidosis

Organs involved	*Siltzbach et al., International study*[1]	*Baughman et al., ACCESS study, USA*[2]	*James et al., UK study*[3]
Lungs	87	95	88
Skin (chronic)	9	15.9	18
Erythema nodosum	17	8.3	34
Lymph nodes	28	11.8	39
Eyes	NA	11.5	27
Liver	NA	8.3	10
Nervous system	4	4.6	9
Cardiac	NA	2.3	3
Calcium abnormality	11	3.7	18
Renal disease	NA	0.7	1

ACCESS, A Case Controlled Etiologic Study of Sarcoidosis.

In a series of 46 patients studied by Bergener and colleagues between 1995 and 2002, 15 (32%) exhibited renal function abnormalities, of whom 10 underwent kidney biopsy; 6 of 10 showed nephrocalcinosis, of whom 2 showed granulomatous interstitial nephritis, 1 interstitial nephritis without granulomas, and 1 immunoglobulin A (IgA) glomerulonephritis. In 2 patients, they found a combination of granulomatous interstitial nephritis with either nephrocalcinosis or with IgA nephritis.[8] The frequency of clinically significant disease remains low. In A Case-Control Etiologic Study of Sarcoidosis (ACCESS), clinical involvement of the kidneys was observed in only 0.7% of patients. Renal involvement may be the initial manifestation of sarcoidosis. It may appear during the course of the illness and follow the onset of the disease after many years. Occasionally, nephrolithiasis is the only presenting feature of sarcoidosis.[9]

A presumptive diagnosis of renal sarcoidosis is justified in cases where typical noncaseating granulomas are found in the kidneys, corticosteroid treatment leads to resolution, and attempts to discover evidence of other causes of granulomatous reaction are unsuccessful. Occasionally, lymphoma and malignancy can produce granulomas.[10] Renal disease in sarcoidosis may be divided into clinical categories as given in table 25-2.

GRANULOMATOUS INTERSTITIAL NEPHRITIS

Although about 20% of patients with sarcoidosis may show granulomas in the kidneys, development of a clinical syndrome of granulomatous interstitial nephritis is unusual. Nevertheless, in a review of 1,010 renal biopsy specimens, Schwartz et al. found only 6 instances of granulomatous interstitial nephritis, all of which were caused by drugs.[11]

GLOMERULONEPHRITIS

The histological changes of focal segmental sclerosis, membranous glomerulonephritis, mesangioproliferative glomerulonephritis, IgA nephropathy, and crescentic glomerulonephritis have been described sporadically. Most such patients have either proteinuria or clinical nephrotic syndrome. Hypertension is frequent, but rarely a serious problem.

Table 25-2 Types of Renal Involvement in Sarcoidosis
Granulomatous interstitial nephritis
Glomerulonephritis
IgA nephropathy (Berger's disease)
Renal cell carcinoma
Granulomatous vasculitis or renal angiitis
Nephrocalcinosis and nephrolithiasis

IgA, immunoglobulin A

Membranous glomerulonephritis (nephropathy) associated with nephritic syndrome is seen in sarcoidosis. Renal biopsy shows membranous nephropathy with or without granulomas, and electron microscopy may reveal typical subepithelial deposits. Corticosteroids are effective.[12-16] Glomerular involvement is rare.

IMMUNOGLOBULIN A NEPHROPATHY (BERGER'S DISEASE) AND GLOMERULAR DISEASE

Membranous and proliferative abnormalities have been described in sarcoidosis. In 1968, Berger and Hinglais first described IgA nephropathy.[25] However, the descriptions from the literature of cases with IgA nephropathy do not reveal precisely the incidence or nature of the relationship between sarcoidosis and IgA nephropathy.[17-20]

INTERSTITIAL NEPHRITIS AND UVEITIS

A curious clinical entity, occurring mainly in women, has been described. It is called tubulointestinal nephritis (TINU) and uveitis syndrome.[21-25] Although its cause is not known, these patients should be evaluated for signs of both sarcoidosis and Sjögren's syndrome (such as xerostomia).[22] Regardless of the cause, this disorder responds to corticosteroid therapy, while lack of treatment may allow progression to chronic renal failure. Recurrent uveitis can occur, but the renal disease is usually cured by the initial course of therapy.[23]

RENAL CARCINOMA AND SARCOIDOSIS

Sarcoid granulomas may be found in regional lymph nodes draining carcinomas or lymphomas (Figure 25-1). Granulomas have also been found in cancerous or

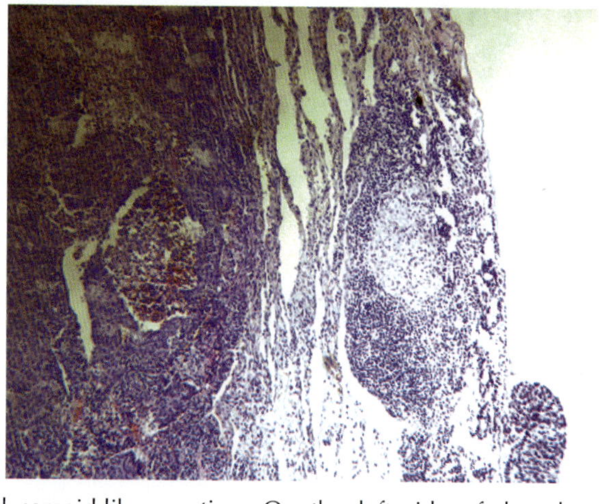

Figure 25-1 Local sarcoid-like reaction. On the left side of the photo one can notice malignant tumor and on the right side " sarcoid like granuloma." Reproduced by the courtesy of Dr Jelena Stojsic, MD, Service of Pathohistology, Clinical Center Serbia, Department of Pathology, Clinic of Pulmonary Diseases and Clinic of Thoracic Surgery.

Table 25-3 Differences between a Non-specific Local Sarcoid Reaction due to Cancer or Trauma and Multisystem Sarcoidosis

	Local sarcoidosis	*Multisystem sarcoidosis*
Number of organs involved	*Usually one*	*More than one*
Age (years)	Any	20–50
Chest radiograph	Usually normal	Abnormal in 90% (most have typical features)
High resolution computed tomography	May suggest tumor, cancer or localized infiltrate	May suggest sarcoidosis
Elevated serum angiotensin converting enzyme	<5 %	>60%
Kveim-Siltzbach test	Negative	Positive in active sarcoidosis
Bronchoalveolar lymphocytes	Absent	Present
Slit-lamp examination	Normal	Positive in 15–20%
Hypercalcemia	May be present in some cancers	Present in more than 10% of sarcoid patient
Whole-body gallium scan	Localized uptake	Multisytem uptake

lymphoma tissue. However, this limited or local granulomatous response should not be confused with multisystem sarcoidosis (Table 25-3). Sporadically, neoplasm, predominantly, breast, renal, or testicular may cause bilateral hilar adenopathy. Rarely, sarcoidosis and neoplasm may coexist but most cases can be separated into a limited granulomatous response or multisystem sarcoidosis by applying strict diagnostic criteria.[12]

GRANULOMATOUS VASCULITIS

Although hyaline deposits in arterial walls occur frequently in sarcoidosis, true obliterative granulomatous involvement of the renal artery is uncommon.

URINARY TRACT DISEASE

Retroperitoneal lymph node involvement, retroperitoneal fibrosis, renal stones, and ureteral involvement may cause ureteral obstruction in sarcoidosis patients (Figure 25-2 and 25-3).[26-29]

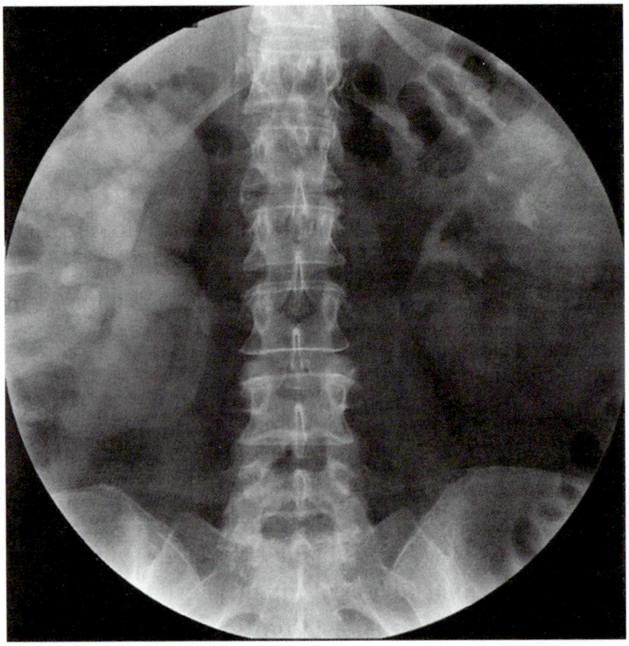

Figure 25-2 Patient with chronic hypercalciuria.

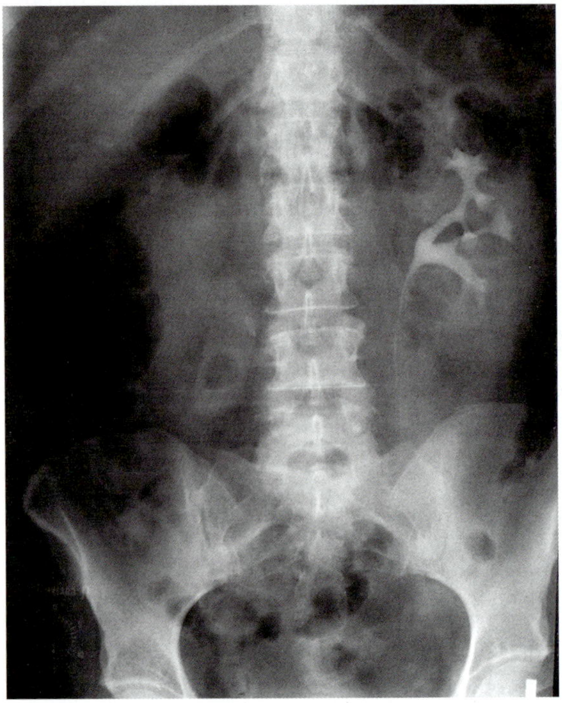

Figure 25-3 Due to renal stone entire loss of function of the right kidney.

REFERENCES

1. Siltzbach L, James D, Neville E, Turiaf J, Battesti JP, Sharma OP, et al. Course and prognosis of sarcoidosis around the world. *Am J Med.* 1974;57:847-52.
2. Baughman RP, Teirstein AS, Judson MA, Rossman MD, Yeager H Jr, Bresnitz EA, et al. Clinical characteristics of patients in a case control study of sarcoidosis (ACCESS). *Am J Respir Cri Care Med.* 2001;164:1885-9.
3. James DG, Neville E, Siltzbach L. A worldwide view of sarcoidosis. *Ann N Y Acad Sci.* 1976;278:321-34.
4. Lower E. Renal sarcoidosis. In: Baughman R, editor. Sarcoidosis, New York: Taylor & Francis; 2006. p. 651.
5. Muther R, McMarron D, Bennett W. Renal manifestations of sarcoidosis. *Arch Intern Med.* 1981;141:643-6.
6. Hagege A, Baglin J, Prinseau J, Goupil A, Laudet J, Fritel D. Sarcoidosis disclosed by renal insufficiency (3 cases). *Sem Hop.* 1983;59:2823-6.
7. Guenel J, Chevet, D. Interstitial nephritis in sarcoidosis. *Presse Med.* 1990;19:1215-7.
8. Bergner R, Hoffmann M, Waldherr R, Uppenkamp M. Frequency of kidney disease in chronic sarcoidosis. *Sarcoidosis Vasc Diffuse Lung Dis.* 2003;20:126-32.
9. Rizzato G, Colombo P. Nephrolithiasis as a presenting feature of chronic sarcoidosis: a prospective study. *Sarcoidosis Vasc Diffuse Lung Dis.* 1996;13:167-72.
10. Sharma OP, Lamb C. Cancer in interstitial lung disease and sarcoidosis. *Curr Opin Pulm Med.* 2003;9:396-401.
11. Schwarz A, Krause PH, Kunzendorf V, Keller F, Distler A. The outcome of interstitial nephritis: risk factors for the transition from acute to chronic interstitial nephritis. *Clin Nephrol.* 2000;54:179-90.
12. Sharma OP. Renal sarcoidosis and hypercalcaemia. *Eur Respir Mon.* 2005;32:220-32.
13. Dimitriades C, Shetty A, Vehaskari M, et al. Membranous nephropathy associated with childhood sarcoidosis. *Pediatr Nephrol.* 1999;13:444-7.
14. Khan IH, Simpson JG, Catto GR, MacLeod AM. Membranous nephropathy and granulomatous nephritis in sarcoidosis. *Nephron.* 1994;66:459-61.
15. Mündlein E, Greten T, Ritz E. Grave's disease and sarcoidosis in a patient with minimal glomerulonephritis. *Nephrol Dial Transplant.* 1996;11:860-2.
16. Parry R, Falk C. Minimal change disease associated with sarcoidosis. *Nephrol Dial Transplant.* 1997;12:2159-60.
17. Taylor J, Ansell I. Sarcoid sensitive nephritis syndrome and renal impairment in a patient with sarcoidosis. *Nephrol Dial Transplant.* 1996;11:355-6.
18. Nishiki M, Murakama Y, Yamane Y, Kato Y. Steroid sensitive nephritic syndrome sarcoidosis and thyroiditis—a new syndrome? *Nephrol Dial Transplant.* 1999;14:2008-10.
19. Schmidt R, Bender F, Change WW, Teba L. Sarcoidosis after renal transplant. *Transplantation.* 1999;68:1420-3.
20. Hamada H, Nagai S, Ono T, Muso E, Nagao T, Shigematsu M, et al. Sarcoidosis complicated with IgA nephropathy. *Sarcoidosis Vasc Diffuse Lung Dis.* 2003;20:69-73.
21. Cacoub P, Deray G, Le Hoang P, Baumelou A, Beaufils H, de Groc F, et al. Idiopathic acute interstitial nephritis associated with anterior uveitis in adults. *Clin Nephrol.* 1989;31:307.
22. Vidal E, Rogues AM, Aldigier JC. The Tinu syndrome or the Sjögren syndrome? *Ann Intern Med.* 1992;116:93.
23. Gafter U, Kalechman Y, Zevin D, Korzets A, Livni E, Klein T, et al. Tubulointerstitial nephritis and uveitis: association with suppressed cellular immunity. *Nephrol Dial Transplant.* 1993;8:821-6.
24. Sessa A, Meroni M, Battini G, Viganò G, Brambilla PL, Paties CT. Acute renal failure due to idiopathic tubulo-intestinal nephritis and uveitis: "TINU syndrome". Case report and review of the literature. *J Nephrol.* 2000;13:377-80.

25. Takemura T, Okada M, Hino S, Fukushima K, Yamamoto S, Miyazato H, et al. Course and outcome of tubulointerstitial nephritis and uveitis syndrome. *Am J Kidney Dis.* 1999;34:1016-21.
26. Fraioli P, Montemurro L, Castrignano L, Rizzato G. Retroperitoneal involvement in sarcoidosis. *Sarcoidosis.* 1990;7:101-5.
27. Godin M, Fillastre JP, Ducastelle T, Hemet J, Morere P, Nouvet G. Sarcoidosis. Retroperitoneal fibrosis, renal arterial involvement, and unilateral focal glomerulosclerosis. *Arch Intern Med.* 1980;140:1240-2.
28. Mariano R, Sussman S. Sarcoidosis of the ureter (letter). *AJR Am J Roentgenol.* 1998;171:1431.
29. Gross KR, Malleson PN, Lirenman DS, McCormick AQ, Petty RE. Vasculopathy with renal artery stenosis in a child with sarcoidosis. *J Pediatr.* 1986;108:724-6.

CHAPTER

26 The Role of Vitamin D in Sarcoidosis

INTRODUCTION

Hypercalcemia and hypercalciuria appear to be important clinical features of sarcoidosis resulting from overproduction of 1,25-dihydroxyvitamin D3 [1,25$(OH)_2D_3$] (calcitriol) by activated macrophages and sarcoidosis granulomas.[1]

Calcium homeostasis is primarily controlled by levels of vitamin D, parathyroid hormone (PTH), and calcitonin, but it is also influenced by thyroid gland and sexual hormones. In sarcoidosis, there is deregulation of these mechanisms, leading to clinically manifested problems.

VITAMIN D AND CALCIUM METABOLISM

Vitamin D insufficiency related to chronic diseases has become a worldwide problem.[2-6] There are 2 forms of vitamin D, vitamin D3 (cholecalciferol), which is produced from the conversion of 7-dehydrocholesterol in the epidermis and dermis in humans, therefore, its nickname "the sunshine vitamin" and vitamin D2 (ergocalciferol) which is produced in mushrooms and yeast. The major source of vitamin D for humans is exposure to sunlight. The efficiency of the conversion of 7-dehydrocholesterol to vitamin D3 is dependent on time of day, season of the year, latitude, skin color, and age. There is little vitamin D that occurs naturally in the food supply. Dietary vitamin D is absorbed from the intestine and circulates in plasma bound to a vitamin D binding protein.[7-8]

In its native form, vitamin D is not biologically active, the active form is 1, 25$(OH)_2D$. Vitamin D is first hydroxylated by the liver to form 25$(OH)_2D$, which is then hydroxylated by the kidney to form 1,25$(OH)_2D$ (calcitriol). 25$(OH)_2D$ has low biological activity, but it is the major form of vitamin D that circulates in the blood stream. Renal synthesis of 1,25$(OH)_2D$ is regulated by plasma PTH together with serum calcium and phosphorus concentrations.[9,10] One of the major biological functions of vitamin D is to maintain calcium homeostasis which impacts on cellular metabolic processes and neuromuscular functions (Figure 26-1). Five biological systems have vitamin D receptors (VDRs) and are responsive to 1,25$(OH)_2D$.

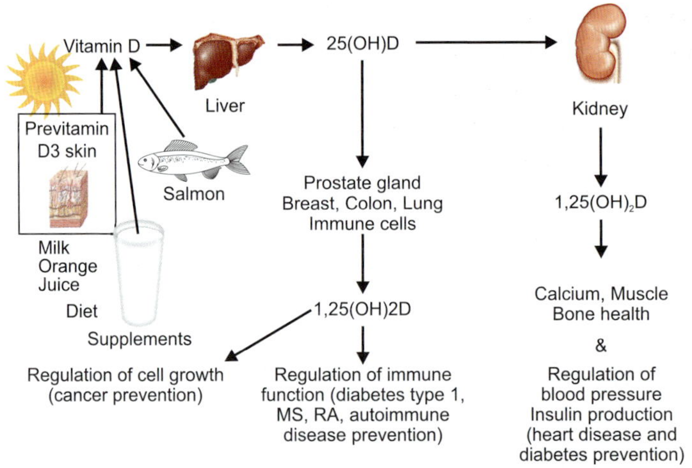

Figure 26-1 The process by which vitamin D is produced and exerts its biological effects is complicated, involving several vitamin D-related molecules. MS, multiple sclerosis; RA, rheumatoid arthritis.[38]

These systems include immune, pancreas, cardiovascular, muscle, and brain; and control of cell cycle. The biological effects of 1,25$(OH)_2$D are diverse. For example, as recently noted, 1,25$(OH)_2$D inhibits PTH secretion and promotes insulin secretion, inhibits adaptive immunity and promotes innate immunity, and inhibits cell proliferation and stimulates their differentiation.[11-15]

Vitamin D was initially thought only to function in calcium homeostasis. However, it has multiple roles in human health, including neuromuscular and immune modulation. Recently, its deficiency is increasingly implicated in many diseases. This discovery has led both popular culture and research to find ways that vitamin D can either treat or prevent many diseases.[16]

Role of 1,25-dihydroxyvitamin D3 in Sarcoidosis

There is indirect evidence that hypovitaminosis D is a risk factor for the development of sarcoidosis. Sarcoidosis is most frequently diagnosed in the winter months, when vitamin D levels nadir.[17]

Moreover, prevalence roughly increases with distance from the equator. Prevalence is particularly high in African-Americans living in the South Eastern United States, a population known to have high rates of vitamin D deficiency.[18]

As increased skin pigmentation is known to reduce the capacity of the skin to convert 7-dehydrocholesterol to previtamin D3, it is reasonable to hypothesize that the more darkly pigmented individuals in these studies had relatively lower levels of vitamin D than lighter skinned individuals in the same location, although serum vitamin D levels are affected by other variables, including dietary choices and food supplementation.[19]

The process of 1-α hydroxylation in the kidney is controlled by PTH and calcitriol. PTH is stimulated by circulation vitamin D metabolites and low levels of ionized calcium to form a bioregulatory loop.[20]

In sarcoidosis, PTH release is inhibited by hypercalcemia and high levels of calcitriol. There are many case reports describing hypoparathyroidism in association with sarcoidosis.[21-23]

The exception, however, is dual pathology as also described in a recent literature, with parathyroid adenoma and coexistent sarcoidosis with granulomas located within the parathyroid adenoma and thyroid gland.[24,25]

Clinical Evidence of the Role of Vitamin D in Sarcoidosis

About 25 years ago, Adams et al. first showed that monocyte/macrophages from sarcoidosis patients synthesized the active form of vitamin-D, $1,25(OH)_2D$ from precursor 25-hydroxyvitamin D(25-OHD).[26]

At the same time, the receptor for $1,25(OH)_2D$ VDR on proliferating lymphocytes was recognized, enlightening another function of D vitamin the function of protecting the inside environment of the host. This is conducted by $1,25(OH)_2D$ cytokine, generated by monocyte-macrophage, interacting with VDR, and modulating the innate immune system to deal with the invading microbes. Increased production of $1,25(OH)_2D$ by activated macrophages is a common finding in many granulomatous inflammation.[27]

The recent review by Drake and Richmond sums up the existing knowledge of hypovitaminosis D as a risk factor for the development of sarcoidosis.[28] The role of vitamin D in inner immunity was strongly supported by the study of Liu et al.,[29] considering another granulomatous inflammatory disease—tuberculosis (TB). These researchers demonstrated that human macrophages increase production of the antimicrobial peptide cathelicidin when stimulated by Toll-like receptor 2/1L, in the presence of $1,25(OH)_2D3$ as occurs in TB infection. Higher cathelicidin levels were in turn shown to improve mycobacteriocidal activity. Since that time, multiple studies show that hypovitaminosis D is a risk factor for the development of active TB.[18,30] Recently, Kanchwala et al. reported that cathelicidin mRNA is present in lower amounts in the bronchoalveolar lavage fluid of sarcoidosis patients; it is much lower in patients with severe sarcoidosis as compared to patients with mild disease, thus both deficiencies of cathelicidin and vitamin D accompany the disease severity in sarcoidosis.[31] The data that support Agerberth et al. study, who asserted that the presence of cathelicidin mRNA in innate immune system may be relevant in persons who are susceptible to vitamin D deficiency.[32]

Thus, the hormonal form of vitamin D seems to possess a role similar to that of cytokines. Calcitriol modulates the cytotoxic and antibody-producing functions of lymphocytes. The action depends on the threshold of VDR expression, and is mediated through inhibition of the T-cell cytokine IL-2.[31] In a study of Kavathia and colleagues,[33] 2 main facts about the role of 1,25(OH)2D in possible predicting the sarcoidosis severity were investigated. These authors found out that elevated serum 1,25$(OH)_2$D levels are positively associated with patients requiring repeated regimes of systemic immunosuppressive therapy or more than 1 year of therapy (patients SCAC 6).[33,34] It is rather possible that the highest level of 1,25$(OH)_2$D leads to hypercalcemia which is the driver of long-term medication use rather than chronic systemic or pulmonary disease.[33]

VITAMIN D AND BEYOND

Completely new field for the discussion might be explored considering neuro-psychological functions in sarcoidosis in relation to serum 25 hydroxyvitamin D levels.[35]

Up to date, no available literature on the topic of the influence of vitamin D in cognitive functions and probably the sensation of fatigue was found related to patients with sarcoidosis. There are studies asserting the receptor for PTH and 1,25(OH)2D in the brain and clinical and experimental data indicating that PTH and vitamin D may affect cerebral function.[36]

How this data can be relayed to patients with sarcoidosis considering depression, fatigue, and cognitive impairments is an opened field for the new researches. No unique rule is available, the evaluation of calcium metabolism and vitamin D in each sarcoidosis patient is obligatory.

MANAGEMENT OF HYPOVITAMINOSIS D IN SARCOIDOSIS

Vitamin D is an important environmental factor in modulating inmate immunity in TB, autoimmunity, multiple sclerosis, and most likely in sarcoidosis.

It is not known whether supplemental vitamin D will prevent or change the course of sarcoidosis. What is known, however, is that symptoms of vitamin D deficiency resemble many of the systemic manifestations of sarcoidosis. It is important to measure serum levels of 25(OH)D and 1,25$(OH)_2$D levels in all patients with sarcoidosis and then correct vitamin D deficiency when found.

The patients with serum 25(OH)D lesser than 30 ng/mL are offered vitamin D supplementation. Sarcoidosis patients who have hypercalcemia should be treated first for their high calcium levels and hen their vitamin D levels be cautiously corrected (Table 26-1).

Table 26-1 Suggested Therapeutic Regime for Vitamin D Supplementation[38]
Ergocalciferol (vitamin D2) 50,000 units weekly for 8 weeks
Serum 25(OH)D levels are rechecked at 8 weeks with a target of 40 ng/mL
Once the targeted serum 25(OH)D levels are achieved, change to cholecalciferol (vitamin D3) and continue at 2,000 IU per day
Levels of 25(OH)D are rechecked every four months

REFERENCES

1. Sharma OP. Renal sarcoidosis and hypercalcaemia. *Eur Respir Mon.* 2005;32:220-232.
2. Kidd MP. Vitamins D and K as pleiotropic nutrients: clinical importance to the skeletal and cardiovascular systems and preliminary evidence for synergy. *Altern Med Rev.* 2010;15:199-222.
3. Melamed ML, Michos ED, Post W, Astor B. 25-hydroxyvitamin D levels and the risk of mortality in the general population. *Arch Intern Med.* 2008;168:1629-37.
4. Dobnig H, Pilz S, Scharnagl H, Renner W, Seelhorst U, Wellnitz B, et al. Independent association of low serum 25-hydroxyvitamin D and 1,25-dihydroxyvitamin D levels with all-cause and cardiovascular mortality. *Arch Intern Med.* 2008;168:1340-9.
5. Peterlik M, Boonen S, Cross HS, Lamberg-Allardt C. Vitamin D and calcium insufficiency-related chronic diseases: an emerging world-wide public health problem. *Int J Environ Res Public Health.* 2009;6:2585-607.
6. Holick MF. The vitamin D deficiency pandemic and consequences for nonskeletal health: mechanisms of action. *Mol Aspects Med.* 2008;29:361-8.
7. Holick MF. Vitamin D deficiency. *N Engl J Med.* 2007;357:266-81.
8. Chung M, Balk EM, Brendel M, Ip S, Lau J, Lee J, et al. Vitamin D and calcium: a systematic review of health outcomes. *Evid Rep Technol Assess (Full Rep).* 2009:1-420.
9. Townsend K, Evans KN, Campbell MJ, Colston KW, Adams JS, Hewison M. Biological actions of extrarenal 25-hydroxyvitamin D-1alpha-hydroxylase and implications for chemoprevention and treatment. *J Steroid Biochem Mol Biol.* 2005;97:103-9.
10. Norman AW. A vitamin D nutritional cornucopia: new insights concerning the serum 25-hydroxyvitamin D status of the US population. *Am J Clin Nutr.* 2008;88:1455-6.
11. Bikle D. Nonclassic actions of vitamin D. *J Clin Endocrinol Metab.* 2009;94:26-34.
12. White JH. Vitamin D signaling, infectious diseases, and regulation of innate immunity. *Infect Immun.* 2008;76:3837-43.
13. Mohr SB. A brief history of vitamin d and cancer prevention. *Ann Epidemiol.* 2009;19:79-83.
14. Dawson-Hughes B. Serum 25-hydroxyvitamin D and functional outcomes in the elderly. *Am J Clin Nutr.* 2008;88:537S-40S.
15. Buell JS, Dawson-Hughes B. Vitamin D and neurocognitive dysfunction: preventing 'D'ecline? *Mol Aspects Med.* 2008;29:415-22.
16. Chu M, Alagiakrishnan K, Sadowski C. The cure of ageing: vitamin D: magic or myth? *Postgrad Med J.* 2010;86:608-16.
17. Newman LS, Rose CS, Maier LA. Sarcoidosis. *N Engl J Med.* 1997;336:1224-35.
18. Ginde AA, Liu MC, Camargo CA. Demographic differences and trends of vitamin D insufficiency in the US population, 1988–2004. *Arch Intern Med.* 2009;169:626-32.
19. Calvo MS, Whiting SJ, Barton CN. Vitamin D intake: a global perspective. *J Nutr.* 2005;135:310-6.
20. Conron M, Young C, Beyon H. Calcium metabolism in sarcoidosis and its clinical implications. *Rheumatology.* 2000;39:707-13.
21. Mitchell T, Stamp T, Jenkins J. Hypercalcemic sarcoidosis in hypoparathyroidism. *Br Med J.* 1983;1:764-5.
22. Karnchanasorn R, Sarikonda M, Aldasouqi S, Gossain VV. Severe hypercalcemia and acute renal failure: an unusual presentation of sarcoidosis. *Case Rep Med.* 2010;2010:423659.
23. Amrein K, Schilcher G, Fahrleitner-Pammer A. Hypercalcaemia in asymptomatic sarcoidosis unmasked by a vitamin D loading dose. *Eur Respir J.* 2011;37:470-1.

24. Chaychi L, Chaidarun S, Golding A, Kinlaw WB, Memoli V, Siegel A. Unusual recurrence of hypercalcemia due to concurrent parathyroid adenoma and parathyroid sarcoidosis with lymph node involvement. *Endocr Pract.* 2010;16:463-7.
25. Balasanthiran A, Sandler B, Amonoo-Kuofi K, Swamy R, Kaniyur S, Kaplan F. Sarcoid granulomas in the parathyroid gland: a case of dual pathology: hypercalcaemia due to a parathyroid adenoma and coexistent sarcoidosis with granulomas located within the parathyroid adenoma and thyroid gland. *Endocrine J.* 2010;57:603-7.
26. Adams J, Hewison M. Update in vitamin D. *J Clin Endocrinol Metab.* 2010;95:471-8.
27. Bhalla AK, Amento EP, Clemens TL, Holick MF, Krane SM. Specific high-affinity receptors for 1,25-dihydroxy vitamin D3 in human peripheral blood mononuclear cells, presence in monocytes and induction in T lymphocytes following activation. *J Clin Endocrinol Metab.* 1983;57:1308-10.
28. Richmond B, Drake W. Vitamin D, innate immunity, and sarcoidosis granulomatous inflammation: insights from mycobacterial research. *Current Opin Pulm Med.* 2010;16:461-4
29. Liu PT, Stenger S, Li H, Wenzel L, Tan BH, Krutzik SR, et al. Toll-like receptor triggering of a vitamin D-mediated human antimicrobial response. *Science.* 2006;311:1770-3.
30. Nnoaham KE, Clarke A. Low serum vitamin D levels and tuberculosis: a systematic review and meta-analysis. *Int J Epidemiol.* 2008;37:113-9.
31. Kanchwala AA, Barna BP, Singh RJ, Culver DA, Malur A, Abraham S, et al. Deficiencies of cathelicidin and vitamin D accompany disease severity in sarcoidosis. *Am J Respir Crit Care Med.* 2009;179:A3997.
32. Agerberth B, Grunewald J, Castaños-Velez E, Olsson B, Jörnvall H, Wigzell H, et al. Antibacterial components in bronchioalveolar lavage fluid from healthy individuals and sarcoidosis patients. *Am J Respir Crit Care Med.* 1999;160:283-90.
34. Kavathia D, Buckley JD, Rao D, Rybicki B, Burke R. Elevated 1, 25-dihydroxyvitamin D levels are associated with protracted treatment in sarcoidosis. *Respir Med.* 2010;104: 564-70.
35. Prasse A, Katic C, Germann M, Buchwald A, Zissel G, Muller-Quernheim J. Phenotyping sarcoidosis from a pulmonary perspective. *Am J Respir Crit Care Med.* 2008;177:330-6.
36. Stechschulte SA, Kirsner RS, Federman DG. Vitamin D: bone and beyond, rationale and recommendations for supplementation. *Am J Med.* 2009;122:793-802.
37. Jorde R, Waterloo K, Saleh F, Haug E, Svartberg J. Neuropsychological function in relation to serum parathyroid hormone and serum 25hydroxyvitamin D levels. *J Neurol.* 2006;253:464-70
38. Sharma OP. Sarcoidosis associated with Vitamin D deficiency? Available from: www.ildcare.eu.

CHAPTER

27 Musculoskeletal Lesions

SKELETAL INVOLVEMENT (ADULTS)

About 25% of patients with sarcoidosis have joint involvement; the true incidence, however, may be difficult to ascertain because some patients may present only with arthritic complaints. Most commonly affected joint areas are knees, ankles, elbows, wrists, and proximal interphalangeal and metacarpophalangeal joints. The affected joints become tender, swollen, and warm to touch. The arthropathies associated with sarcoidosis can be divided into either acute or chronic, with the latter having the potential to be aggressive and at times cause deformities of the joints.[1]

Acute arthritis may present in isolation or as part of Lofgren's syndrome (Figure 27-1).[2] The chronic arthritis, unlike the acute arthropathy of sarcoid, is frequently associated with chest radiographic findings of parenchymal lung disease. Joint effusions are common, but are less frequent in large joints. Synovial joint biopsy may or may not show the classic noncaseating granulomas (Figure 27-2).[3,4] Sarcoidosis bone lesions are characterized by:

- Bilateral distribution
- The site of origin (cortical, preservation of the periosteum)

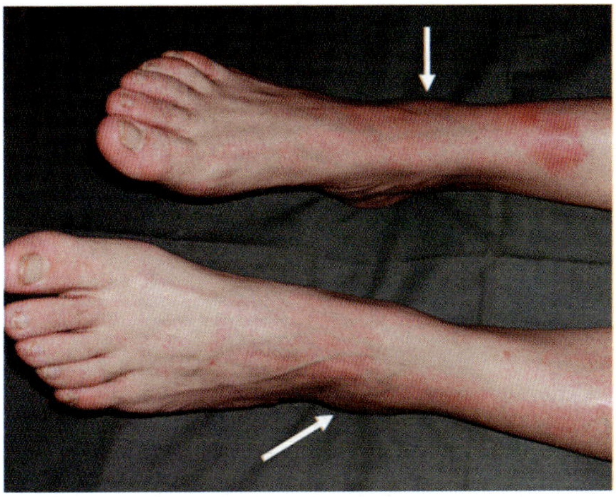

Figure 27-1 Acute arthritis as part of Lofgren's syndrome.

- Location (hands and feet)
- Position (usually the ends of the affected bones)
- The shape (cystic or lacelike with minimal disturbance of the nearby soft tissues).

SKELETAL INVOLVEMENT (CHILDREN)

Sarcoid arthropathy in children is relatively rare, but must be considered if an infant or a child develops fever and multiple joint swellings. Most reported childhood cases of sarcoid arthritis occur later in the childhood and preadolescence years. In this age group, sarcoidosis usually presents with the triad of uveitis, rash, and arthritis. The characteristic erythematous macular rash is widespread and prominent on flexor surfaces. Joints of both upper and lower extremities can be affected with frequent effusions. Joint erosions are absent.[5] Sarcoidosis in a 7-month old infant has been observed.[6]

MUSCLE INVOLVEMENT

Muscle involvement is frequently encountered on histopathological examinations, yet clinically, the patients are asymptomatic. The symptoms are decreased exercise tolerance, weakness, pain or ache, or muscle nodules. There are 3 different clinical types of sarcoid myopathies: (i) the acute type which is common, presents with proximal muscle weakness, (ii) the chronic type, presents with muscle wasting and weakness, and rarely (iii) the nodular type. Creatinine kinase levels may or

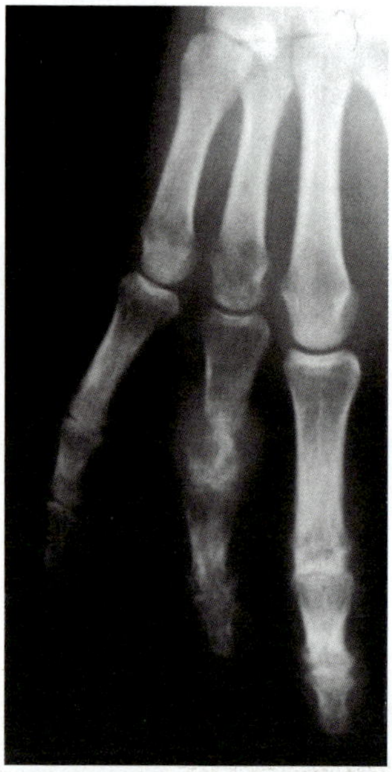

Figure 27-2 Lytic bone lesion with destruction and soft tissue swelling. Biopsy revealed sarcoidosis.

Table 27-1 Differences between Myopathy due to Sarcoidosis and due to Steroids[8]

	Steroid-induced myopathy	*Sarcoid myopathy*
Clinical features	Myalgia; proximal weakness, especially legs	Myalgia; weakness: proximal more than distal; sometimes palpable nodules, contractures or cramp
Creatine kinase	Mostly normal	Sometimes elevated
Frequency	Low: 2–21% in all patients receiving steroids	50% of sarcoidosis patients have muscle granulomas, often asymptomatic
Electromyography	Low amplitude MUPs of short duration	Fibrillations and positive sharp waves; low amplitude MUPs of short duration
Biopsy	Type-2 fiber atrophy	Myositis; nodular myositis

MUP, motor unit potential.

may not be elevated in these patients. Nodular myopathy is often painful. On magnetic resonance imaging, the nodules can be mistaken for soft tissue tumors. Muscle biopsies show the characteristic sarcoid granulomas in up to 50% of sarcoid myopathic patients.[7]

It is very important for the clinicians to distinguish sarcoid myopathy from steroid induced myopathy (Table 27-1).[8]

REFERENCES

1. Visser H, Vos K, Zanelli E, Verduyn W, Schreuder GM, Speyer I, et al. Sarcoid arthritis: clinical characteristics, diagnostic aspects, and risk factors. *Ann Rheum Dis.* 2002;61:499-504.
2. Mañá J, Gómez-Vaquero C, Montero A, Salazar A, Marcoval J, Valverde J, et al. Löfgren's syndrome revisited: a study of 186 patients. *Am J Med.* 1999;107:240-5.
3. Grigor RR, Hughes GR. Chronic sarcoid arthritis. *Br Med J.* 1976;2:1044.
4. Torralba KD, Quismorio FP Jr. Sarcoid arthritis: a review of clinical features, pathology and therapy. *Sarcoidosis Vasc Diffuse Lung Dis.* 2003;20:95-103.
5. Pattishall EN, Strope GL, Spinola SM, Denny EL. Childhood sarcoidosis. *J Pediatr.* 1986; 108:169-77.
6. Kendig EL Jr. Sarcoidosis in children: personal observations on age distribution. *Pediatric Pulmonol.* 1989;6:69-70.
7. Ibrahim F, Sharma O. Clinical Manifestations of Sarcoidosis. In: Sharma OP, editor. Interstitial lung disease. New Delhi: Jaypee Medical Publishers Ltd.; 2011. p. 469-82.
8. Hoitsma E, Sharma OP. Neurosarcoidosis. In: Drent M, Costabel U, editors. Sarcoidosis (European Respiratory Monograph). European Respiratory Society; 2005. p. 164-87.

CHAPTER

28 Sarcoidosis and Common Variable Immunodeficiency

INCIDENCE

Most physicians taking care of sarcoidosis patients have encountered the occurrence of immune deficiency syndromes in sarcoidosis. The immune deficiency is discovered when these patients develop recurrent infections in the lungs, sinuses, and skin. Occasionally, presence of an autoimmune disease associated with sarcoidosis draws attention to the existence of immunodeficiency.[1] Conversely, the common variable immunodeficiency (CVID) patients develop multisystem granulomas typical of sarcoidosis.[2]

CLINICAL FEATURES

Persistent variable cough with expectoration are symptoms that particularly plague these patients. Initially, the symptoms are neither recognized nor adequately investigated because sarcoidosis is not commonly appreciated as primary immunodeficiency. Furthermore, the immunodeficiency often presents, for the first time in childhood, the age group that is not affected by sarcoidosis. Finally, the diagnosis is not considered because the symptoms can be wrongly attributed to other common adult conditions including asthma, chronic obstructive pulmonary disease, bronchiectasis, allergies, and gastroesophageal reflux diseases related to lung disease.[3]

COMMON VARIABLE IMMUNODEFICIENCY IN SARCOIDOSIS

Patients with sarcoidosis who have chronic cough and recurrent infections should be evaluated for CVID. Patients with CVID in whom sarcoidosis develops present a higher prevalence of recurrent infections, thrombocytopenia, and splenic involvement. Steroids, in most cases subdue adenopathy and splenic enlargement, improve uveitis, lower serum alkaline phosphatase, and reverse hematologic abnormalities. The underlying mechanism responsible for the association of these 2 disorders in the same patient remains obscure. However, as more patients are identified, it may be possible to gain a better understanding of the immunologic defect responsible for the dual presentation of these 2 relatively uncommon diseases.

SARCOIDOSIS IN COMMON VARIABLE IMMUNODEFICIENCY

The occurrence of systemic sarcoidosis in combination with CVID has been described in only a small number of patients. In these patients, lymphadenopathy, mild to moderate pulmonary involvement, and hepatosplenomegaly are common. In 1971, an adult Caucasian woman with hypogammaglobulinema, depression of delayed type-hypersensitivity, and widespread granuloma formation in lymph nodes and liver was reported (Figures 28-1 and 28-2). The chest X-ray film showed nondiagnostic diffuse infiltration and areas of linear atelectasis.[4] Fasano et al. reported 8 cases of sarcoidosis among their 80 patients with CVID. They reviewed the literature and found 22 other cases of the combined occurrence. The authors emphasized that sarcoidosis should be considered in a patient with CVID who presents with clinical, radiographic, laboratory, and biopsy findings consistent with sarcoidosis.[5] Patients with CVID can develop noncaseating granulomas in the lymphoid or solid organs, including the lungs, lymph nodes, liver, intestine, spleen, brain, or skin. It is estimated that 8–20% of CVID patients have some form of granulomatous disease, although the prevalence is probably underappreciated since most tissues are not biopsied. The multisystem granuloma formation in CVID can resemble multisystem sarcoidosis.

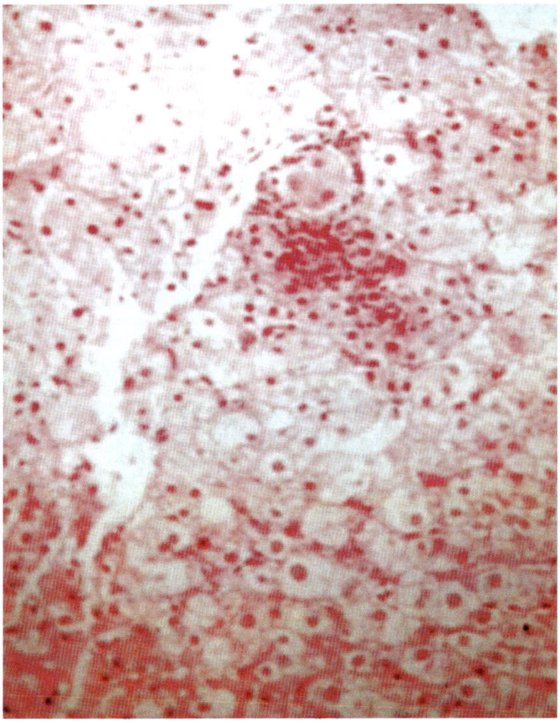

Figure 28-1 Lymph node biopsy in the same patient showing a dense granuloma with mixed cell population (H&Ex100).[4]

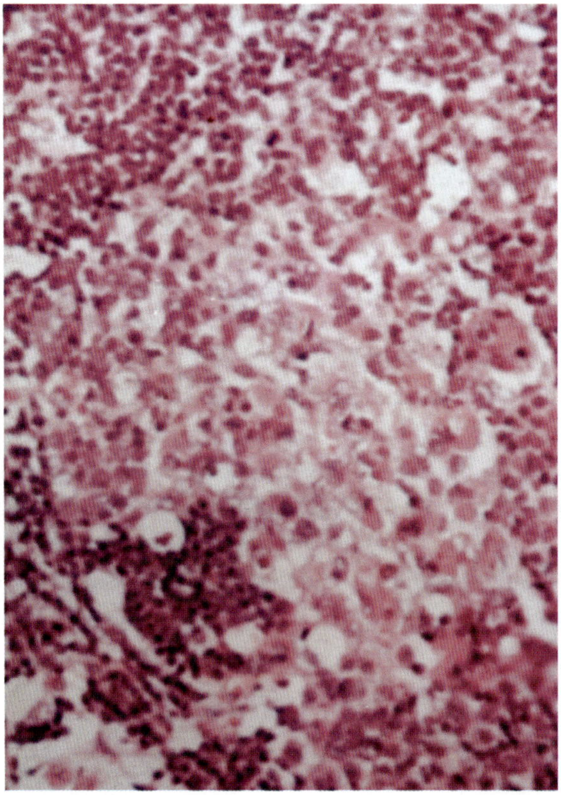

Figure 28-2 Granulomatous inflammation in patient with hypogammaglobulinemia. Liver biopsy in patient with hypogammaglobulinemia. Biopsy shows a collection of early granulomatous response (HEx50).[4]

Common presentations include lymphadenopathy, splenomegaly, and pulmonary symptoms. Severe and rapidly progressive pulmonary fibrosis in combination with a severe defect of the cellular and humoral immune system has not been described. Many patients with granulomatous infiltration of the liver and lungs have variable elevations in angiotensin converting enzyme levels.[6]

PATHOGENESIS

The pathogenesis of noncaseating granulomas in CVID is uncertain. An unusual tumor necrosis factor (TNF) polymorphism has been found in increased numbers, but any effect on TNF levels or usage has not been examined. An abnormal CD8+ T cell response to cytomegalovirus has also been detected in patients with CVID and inflammatory disease. There was a progressively reduced lymphocyte proliferation in response to T cell mitogens, while proliferation after specific interleukin (IL)-2 stimulation was normal. A Th1 lymphocyte-subset-like profile might thus play a role in the pathogenesis and might form the connecting link.

Autoimmune conditions are diagnosed in almost one-quarter of CVID patients. A review of 326 CVID patients found that 11% had a history of immune thrombocytopenic purpura, autoimmune hemolytic anemia, or Evans' syndrome. Approximately one-half of these developed hematologic autoimmune disease before or concurrent with the diagnosis of CVID.

INVESTIGATIONS

Neutropenia, lymphopenia, and low serum globulin may be subtle and nonspecific manifestations of immunodeficiency. The most common immunodeficiency syndromes can be identified by easily available tests. The acronym FISH (full blood count, immunoglobulins, serum complement C3/C4) is a mnemonic for the common first line investigation. A new combination of severe immunodeficiency, and sarcoidosis, and cleft-palate has been reported.[7,8]

CONCLUSION

Association of sarcoidosis and immune efficiency syndromes is more frequent than has been appreciated in the past either by practicing physicians or pulmonary specialists. Sarcoidosis is an important entity among the patients with CVID who exhibit clinical, radiographic, laboratory, and biopsy findings compatible with sarcoidosis. Conversely, the diagnosis of CVID should be considered in patients with sarcoidosis who do not exhibit hypergammaglobulinemia, the characteristic biochemical abnormality of sarcoidosis, and who have a history of recurrent infections of sinuses, lungs, or skin.

REFERENCES

1. Brandt D, Gershwin ME. Common variable immunodeficiency (CVID) and autoimmunity. *Autoimmun Rev*. 2006;5:465-70.
2. Artac H, Bozkurt B, Talim B, Reisil I. Sarcoid-like granulomas and common variable immunodeficiency. *Rheumatol Int*. 2009:30:109-12.
3. Javidan-Nejad C, Bhalla S. Bronchiectasis (review). *Radiol Clin North Am*. 2009;47:289-306.
4. Sharma OP, James DG. Hypogammaglobulinemia, depression of delayed-type hypersensitivity, and granuloma formation. *Amer Rev Respir Dis*. 1971;104:228-31.
5. Fasano MB, Sullivan KE, Sarpong SB, Wood RA, Jones SM, Lederman HM, et al. Sarcoidosis and common variable immunodeficiency. Report of 8 cases and review of the literature. *Medicine (Baltimore)*. 1996;75;251-61.
6. Sutor G, Fabel H. Sarcoidosis and common variable immunodeficiency: a case of malignant course of sarcoidosis in conjunction with severe impairment of cellular and humoral immune system. *Respiration*. 2000;67:204-8.
7. Huisoon AP, Krishna MT. Does this patient have immunodeficiency? *Clin Med*. 2011; 11:380-4.
8. Leibla A, Apter S, Leibla M, Thaler M, Grossman E. Acute respiratory failure in a patient with sarcoidosis and immunodeficiency: an unusual presentation and a complicated course. *Lung*. 2004;182:73-7.

CHAPTER

29 Cancer and Sarcoidosis

INCIDENCE

A 38-year-old woman developed left upper quadrant abdominal fullness. She had no fever, chills, anorexia, night-sweats, or weight loss. Physical examination showed small, nontender, movable lymph nodes in the posterior cervical triangles on both sides and a nontender enlarged spleen. She had mild anemia and eosinophilia. A cervical lymph node biopsy showed noncaseating granulomas consistent with the diagnosis of sarcoidosis. She was treated with prednisone, but the drug was discontinued because of severe side effects. Methotrexate was given; it caused her to loose hair. Infliximab was also given. After 6 infusions of 5 mg/kg body weight each, she came down with pneumonia. She was treated successfully for it, but it was decide, to discontinue infliximab. She developed night sweats and fatigue and her spleen increased to more than 6 cm below the left coastal margin. A splenic biopsy showed features of Hodgkin's disease. The following diagnostic possibilities seem reasonable to explain her clinical course:

- The patient had both sarcoidosis and lymphoma. The finding of noncaseating granuloma in the lymph nodes was a "red-herring" that obscured and delayed the diagnosis of lymphoma
- The patient had sarcoidosis first and then developed lymphoma later, but it would be unusual because in patients who have both illnesses, lymphoma appears first followed by sarcoidosis months and years later
- The patient had sarcoidosis and infliximab treatment in some manner induced the development of lymphoma. There is no good evidence in literature to support this hypothesis.

WHAT IS THE RELATIONSHIP BETWEEN SARCOIDOSIS AND CANCER/LYMPHOMA?

Data analysis from a 10 year study of 2,544 patients from the Danish Sarcoidosis Registry[1] discovered 48 patients with sarcoidosis who had cancer. Out of this group, lung cancer occurred 3 times frequently than in general population, while patients with sarcoidosis who had lymphoma occurred 11 times more than in general population.

Romer,[2] reanalyzing the same cohort of sarcoidosis patients, reported that 29% of patients were misdiagnosed with sarcoidosis.

However, in a study of Seersholm and colleagues,[3] the authors revealed no link between cancer and sarcoidosis during a long period of follow-up of a cohort of 254 patients with pulmonary sarcoidosis. The patients were followed for 25 years on average.

CLINICAL SIGNIFICANCE

The precise mechanism of sarcoidosis-cancer syndrome is not clear. There are several possible scenarios of coexistence of malignancy and sarcoidosis:

- In patients with hematological malignancies (sarcoidosis-lymphoma syndrome)
- In sarcoidosis patients who develop solid tumors
- Paraneoplastic sarcoidosis
- Antineoplastic treatment associated sarcoidosis
- Sarcoid-like reactions and malignancy

Sarcoidosis-lymphoma Syndrome

The term was first coined by Brincker[4] in 1986, describing the clinical appearance of sarcoidosis that precedes the diagnosis of lymphoma. Besides Hodgkin's disease, the most frequently associated other lymphoproliferative diseases that may occur include, i.e., non-Hodgkin lymphoma, myeloma, chronic myelogenous leukemia, and chronic lymphocitic leukemia.[1,4-10]

In a 10 year study of 2,544 patients with pulmonary sarcoidosis, the authors found the occurrence of malignant lymphoma 11 times more frequently in sarcoidosis population, and hypothesized that the coexistence of sarcoidosis and lymphoproliferative disease, i.e., lymphoma developed due to an immunological response, most likely increased mitotic activity of the lymphocytes.[1]

Sarcoidosis and Solid Tumors

There is an increased incidence of solid tumors and sarcoidosis. Evidence based studies[6,11-13] revealed that organs affected with sarcoidosis have been at increased risk of developing solid tumors (i.e., hapatocellular carcinoma of the liver, melanoma, and nonmelanoma skin malignancy.[3,6,12-17]

In patients with active pulmonary sarcoidosis, an increased incidence of developing lung cancer was observed.[11,18,19] There are 2 possible explanations for this fact—either solid tumor can represent "scar cancer", developing at the site of previous sarcoid nodules of the lung or the immunological abnormalities in sarcoidosis that lead to the decreased defense against oncogenic viruses.[13,15,18,19]

An increased risk of sarcoidosis, however, was described in a literature in patients with testicular carcinoma, cervical cancer, and cancer of the uterus.[3,14,15,20-24]

Paraneoplastic Sarcoidosis

Diagnosis of paraneoplastic sarcoidosis in patients with solid tumors occurs at the same time with the diagnosis of malignancy (often within the same year); most frequently in patients with breast cancer and kidney.[25,26]

Antineoplastic Therapy Associated Sarcoidosis

This form of sarcoidosis occurs after antineoplastic therapy in oncological patients with previously undiagnosed sarcoidosis. This form of sarcoidosis is described most frequently in patients with Hodgkin's disease, non-Hodgkin lymphoma,[27] and multiple myeloma, but it has also been reported in patients with solid tumors treated with methotrexate (osteosarcoma), alpha interferon (melanoma, renal cell carcinoma), and also noted in patients treated with cisplatin.[28-31]

Sarcoid-like Reaction and Malignancy

Sarcoid-like reactions have been described usually in the lymph nodes draining the cancer. However, sarcoid-like reaction may also occur in the stroma, the organ of tumor origin, and tissues distant from the organ involved with primary cancer like spleen, bone marrow, and skin.[32-36]

Most frequently, sarcoid-like reactions are noticed in patients with Hodgkin's disease (13.8%), non-Hodgkin's (7.3%), and in patients with carcinomas (4.4%).[36,37]

It has been postulated that the main mechanism of sarcoid-like reaction is the host's immune response (a local T-cell mediated immune response), in the draining lymph nodes, where soluble antigenic tumor factors (tumor cells or products of tumor necrosis) are transported by lymphatic vessels.[37,38]

It is most important to differentiate sarcoid-like reactions from noncaseating granulomas in systemic sarcoidosis (Table 29-1).[39-41]

Table 29-1 Difference between a Local Sarcoid Reaction and Systemic Sarcoidosis

Features	*Local sarcoid reaction*	*Multisystem sarcoidosis*
Organ(s) involved	Single	Multiorgan
Age	Any	Middle age
Associated disease	Malignancy	None
Pathogenesis	May be local immune response	Unknown
Chest radiograph	Normal	Abnormal
Delayed hypersensitivity	May be normal	Depressed
Elevated serum ACE	Absent	60% of the patients
Hyperglobulinemia	Absent	Present in about one third of the patients
BAL lymphocytosis	Absent/present in lymphoma	Present
Slit lamp examination	Normal	Abnormal in15–20%
Hypercalcemia	Absent/can be present in cancer patients	10% of the patients
Gallium/PET body scan	Localized uptake	Multisystem uptake

ACE, angiotensin-converting enzyme; BAL, bronchoalveolar lavage; PET positron emission tomography.

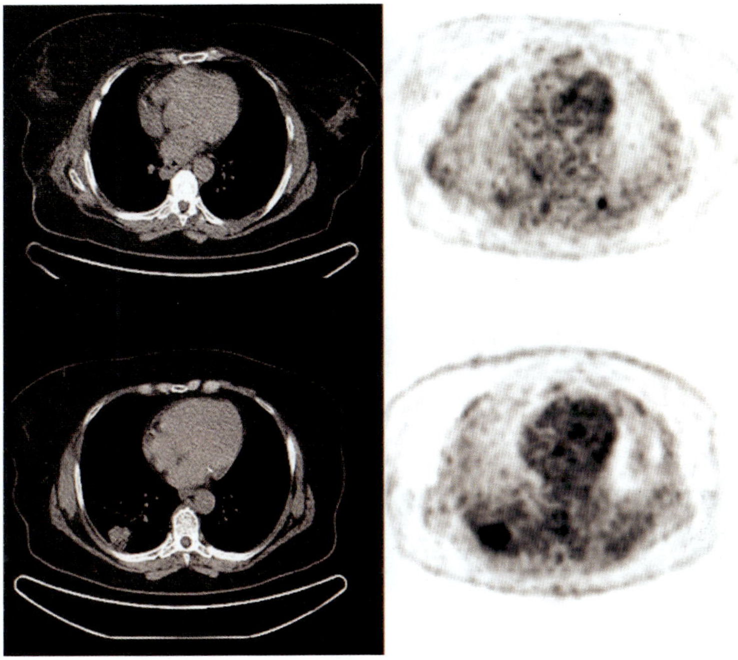

Figure 29-1 Position emission tomography scan, July 2011, detecting lung new growth in the low lobe right.

Of note, the presence of sarcoid-like reactions has been shown to signify positive prognosis especially in patients with Hodgkin's disease and gastric cancer.[34]

The awareness of sarcoid-cancer coexistence (sarcoid-cancer syndrome) has also raised the need for prompt diagnostic procedures, because early and accurate diagnosis improves the possibility of successful therapy.

Figure 29-1 demonstrates lung cancer in sarcoidosis patient treated with methotrexate. Although described in patients with rheumatoid arthritis after long-term treatment with methotrexate,[28] lung malignancy has not been described in sarcoidosis patients who were also treated with methotrexate. The patient had biopsy positive lung sarcoidosis for years. The treatment with methotrexate due to chronic form of pulmonary sarcoidosis lasted for 5 years. In the year 2011 July, she came with terrible dry cough and chest pain (area of the lower part of her right lung). Positron emission tomography (PET) scan discovered very high standardized uptake max value susceptible for malignancy.

Bronchoscopy revealed lung tumor of the right low lobe—large squamous cell lung cancer. The operation was performed—right lobectomy (Figure 29-2).

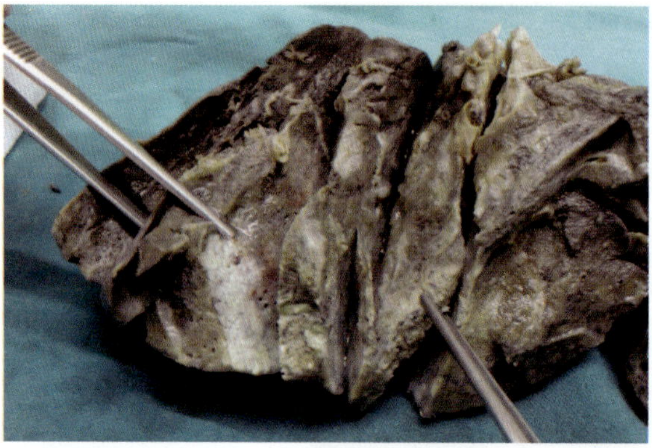

Figure 29-2 Lower lobe of the right lung with tumor.

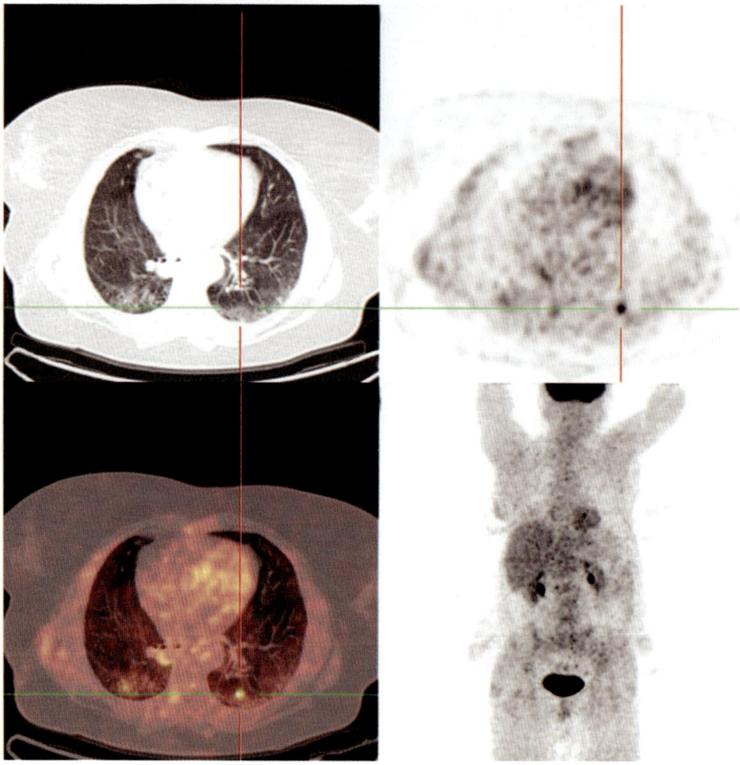

Figure 29-3 Position emission tomography scan of the same patient December 2011, 5 months after the operation.

After the operation, control PET scan revealed no signs of the tumor (Figure 29-3). Her sarcoidosis relapsed after the operation, but this time she was treated with steroid therapy.

REFERENCES

1. Brincker H, Wilbek E. The incidence of malignant tumors in patients with sarcoidosis. *Ugeskr Laeger.* 1974;136:2192-5.
2. Romer F. Sarcoidosis and cancer: a critical review. In Eighth International Conference on Sarcoidosis and Other Granulomatous Diseases. Cardiff, Wales: Alpha Omega; 1980. p. 567-71.
3. Seersholm N, Vestbo J, Viskum K. Risks of malignant neoplasm in patients with pulmonary sarcoidosis. *Thorax.* 1997;52:892-4.
4. Brincker H. The sarcoidosis-lymphoma syndrome. *Br J Cancer.* 1986;54:467-73.
5. Oliwiecki S, Kingston T, Kotecha B, Rothera MP. Sarcoidosis lymphoma syndrome. *J Royal Soc Med.* 1992;85:176-7.
6. Brincker H, Wilbek E. The incidence of malignant tumours in patients with respiratory sarcoidosis. *Br J Cancer.* 1974;29:247-51.
7. Karakantza M, Matutes E, MacLennan K, O'Connor NTJ, Srivastava PC, Catovsky D. Association between sarcoidosis and lymphoma revisited. *J Clin Pathol.* 1996;49:208-12.
8. Ryan PJ, Stableforth P, McLeod DT. Co-existing conjunctival non-Hodgkin's lymphoma and pulmonary sarcoidosis. *Thorax.* 1996;51:444-5.
9. Simsek S, van Leuven F, Bronsveld W, Ooms GH, Groeneveld ABJ, de Graaff CS. Unusual association of Hodgkin's disease and sarcoidosis. *J Med.* 2002;60:438-40.
10. Serratrice J, Granel B, Swiader L, Disdier P, Weiller-Merli C, Lepidi H, et al. Sarcoidosis preceding chronic myelomonocytic leukemia: report of two cases. *Dermatology.* 2002; 205:409-12.
11. Brincker H. Sarcoidosis and malignancy. *Chest.* 1995;108:1472-4.
12. Brincker H. Solid tumors preceding or following sarcoidosis. *Med Pediatr Oncol.* 1987;15:82-8.
13. Reich JM. Malignant neoplasms in pulmonary sarcoidosis. *Thorax.* 1998;53:625-6.
14. Romer FK, Hommelgaard P, Schou G. Sarcoidosis and cancer revisited: a long-term follow-up study of 555 Danish sarcoidosis patients. *Eur Respir J.* 1998;12:906-12.
15. Askling J, Grunewald J, Eklund A, Hillerdal G, Ekbom A. Increased risk for cancer following sarcoidosis. *Am J Respir Crit Care Med.* 1999;160:1668-72.
16. Chalasani P, Vohra M, Sheagren JN. An association of sarcoidosis with hepatocellular carcinoma. *Ann Oncol.* 2005;16:1714-5.
17. McLoone NM, McKenna K, Edgar D, Walsh M, Bingham A. Merkel cell carcinoma in a patient with chronic sarcoidosis. *Clin Exp Dermatol.* 2005;30:580-2.
18. Yanagawa H, Goto H, Maniwa K, et al. A case of respectable lung adenocarcinoma associated with sarcoidosis. *Med Oncol.* 1999;16:216-20.
19. Yamasawa H, Ishii Y, Kitamura S. Concurrence of sarcoidosis and lung cancer: a report of four cases. *Respiration.* 2000;67:90-3.
20. de Hemricourt E, de Boeck K, Hilte F, Abib A, Kockx M, Vandevivere J, et al. Sarcoidosis and sarcoid-like reaction following Hodgkin's disease. Report of two cases. *Mol Imaging Biol.* 2003;5:15-9.
21. Reich JM, Mullooly JP, Johnson RE. Linkage analysis of malignancy associated sarcoidosis. *Chest.* 1995;107:605-13.
22. Alliot C, Barrios M, Desplechain C. Multisystem sarcoidosis and carcinoma of the uterine cervix: an unusual association. *Int J Gynecol Cancer.* 2001;11:323-5.
23. Muggia FM, Conti PS. Seminoma and sarcoidosis: a cause for false positive mediastinal uptake in PET? *Ann Oncol.* 1998;9:924.

24. Rayson D, Burch PA, Richardson RL. Sarcoidosis and testicular carcinoma. *Cancer.* 1998;83:337-43.
25. Lower EE, Hawkins HH, Baughman RP. Breast disease in sarcoidosis. *Sarcoidosis Vasc Diffuse Lung Dis.* 2001;18:301-6.
26. Logan TF, Bensadoun ES. Increased disease activity in a patient with sarcoidosis after high dose interleukin 2 treatment for metastatic renal cancer. *Thorax.* 2005;60:610-1.
27. Kornacker M, Kraemer A, Leo E,Ho AD. Occurrence of sarcoidosis subsequent to chemotherapy for non-Hodgkin's lymphoma: report of two cases. *Ann Hematol.* 2002: 81:103-5.
28. Massaguer S, Sanchez M, Castel T. Mediastinal sarcoidosis induced by high-dose alpha-2-interferon therapy in a patient with malignant melanoma. *Eur Radiol.* 2004;14:1716-7.
29. Sybert A, Butler TP. Sarcoidosis following adjuvant high-dose methotrexate therapy for osteosarcoma. *Arch Intern Med.* 1978;138:488-9.
30. Ravenel JG, McAdams HP, Plankeel JF, Butnor KJ, Sporn TA. Sarcoidosis induced by interferon therapy. Case report. *AJR Am J. Roentgenol.* 2001;177:199-201.
31. Abdi EA, Nguyen GK, Ludwig RN, Dickout WJ. Pulmonary sarcoidosis following interferon therapy for advanced renal cell carcinoma. *Cancer.* 1987;59:896-900.
32. Kurata A, Terado Y, Schulz A, Fujioka Y, Franke FE. Inflammatory cells in the formation of tumor-related sarcoid reactions. *Hum Pathol.* 2005;36:546-54.
33. Pandha HS, Griffiths H,Waxman J. Sarcoidosis and cancer. *Clin Oncol (R Coll Radiol).* 1995;7:277-8.
34. Sacks EL, Donaldson SS, Gordon J, Dorfman RF. Epithelioid granulomas associated with Hodgkin's disease. Clinical correlation in 55 previously untreated patients. *Cancer.* 1978;41:562-7.
35. Berg van den, Fickers M, Theunissen P, van Noord JA. Pulmonary sarcoid-like granulomata in a patient treated for extrapulmonary Hodgkin's disease. *Respiration.* 1997;64:114-7.
36. Brincker H. Sarcoid reactions and sarcoidosis in Hodgkin's disease and other malignant lymphomata. *Br J Cancer.* 1972;26:120-8.
37. Brincker H. Sarcoid reactions in malignant tumours. *Cancer Treat Rev.* 1986;13:147-56.
38. Bassler R, Birke F. Histopathology of tumour associated sarcoid-like stromal reaction in breast cancer. An analysis of 5 cases with immunohistochemical investigations. *Virchows Arch A Pathol Anat Histopathol.* 1988;412:231-9.
39. Kurata A, Takayama N, Terado Y, Hirano K, Yokoyama K, Fujioka Y. Sarcoidal granulomas in the spleen associated with multiple carcinomas. *Sarcoidosis Vasc Diffuse Lung Dis.* 2010;27:153-9.
40. Kurata A, Terado Y, Schulz A, Fujioka Y, Franke FE. Inflammatory cells in the formation of tumor-related sarcoid reactions. *Hum Pathol.* 2005;36:546-54.
41. Pandha HS, Griffiths H, Waxman J. Sarcoidosis and cancer. *Clin Oncol.* 1995;7:277-8.

CHAPTER

30 Sarcoidosis or/and Tuberculosis Comorbidity or the Consequence?

INTRODUCTION

Nowadays, even with the scientific progress of the 21st century, distinguishing between sarcoidosis and tuberculosis (TB) can be a challenge. If we avoid the classic definition of sarcoidosis and put emphasis on the main clinical manifestations of these 2 diseases, the conclusions might be the following:

- The main manifestations of both diseases are in the lungs, and are associated with systemic symptoms, such as fever, malaise, anorexia, and weight loss[1,2]
- Both diseases can affect the same organs (i.e., lymph nodes, liver, spleen, musculoskeletal system, skin, eye, central nervous system, and so on)
- Both can produce granuloma, which may be noncaseating in sarcoidosis as well as in TB.[1,2]

At the end of the 19th century when sarcoidosis was described for the first time, the disease was assumed to be a variation of TB.

Sarcoidosis is a granulomatous disease. Many agents are known as possible cause of granulomas among which infection is the most common. These include TB and fungal infections, such as histoplasmosis.

Thus, most physicians associate a granulomatous response with an infectious cause. TB has frequently been quoted as a possible cause of sarcoidosis.[3] Some investigators found an association between the prevalence of TB and the prevalence of sarcoidosis.[4] The other studies, however, demonstrated clearly that sarcoidosis was not associated with active tuberculous infection.[5,6]

The diagnosis of sarcoidosis (versus TB) is usually supported by the clinical picture, the negative purified protein derivative (PPD) test, the noncaseating granuloma, the absence of *Mycobacterium tuberculosis*, and an excellent response to corticosteroids. Is the positive polymerase chain reaction (PCR) examination of the biopsy sample(s) sufficient enough to rule out the diagnosis of sarcoidosis?

Several studies have shown the presence of *Mycobacterium* DNA in sarcoid granuloma, suggesting previous exposure to *Mycobacterium*, which might have induced a granulomatous reaction.[7]

The key to the diagnosis of TB is a high degree of awareness. The laboratory diagnosis is based on several methods, such as direct microscopy, tissue culture, and PCR-based nucleic acid amplification techniques. Although direct microscopy has low sensitivity (about 65%), tissue culture is a "gold standard" for diagnosis. However, it requires 4–6 weeks before growth is detected.[8]

The biopsy sample tissue has been explored with various molecular techniques, i.e., PCR. However, this technique has certain faults, including use of nonspecific primers and failure to use adequate controls. Using more severe criteria, others have not verified that *M. tuberculosis* was present in the tissue of most patients with sarcoidosis.[9] The principal advantage of PCR methods is that they provide a rapid diagnosis with extremely high sensitivity of 97–100% and specificity of 90–100% for any form of TB infection (active, treated, or asymptomatic).[10] On the other hand, the positive PCR test does not necessarily imply active TB, the specificity for the active form being only 70%.[11,12]

Recent innovative blood tests that measure the cell-mediated immune response of TB-infected individuals like quantiferon-TB test are highly specific for detecting *M. tuberculosis* infection. However, even the quantiferon-TB gold test was positive in 3.3% of Japanese sarcoidosis patients.[13]

By following individual patients, investigators found that the tuberculin skin test could go from positive, indicating TB infection, to negative, indicating anergy from sarcoidosis.[6]

It is also believed that corticosteroid treatment might contribute to the reactivation (exacerbation) of TB,[14] although the risk of corticosteroid treatment in patients with previous exposure to TB is probably lower than is generally believed.[15,16]

Rarely, sarcoidosis and TB might coexist in the same patient, although the cases are limited to a couple of case reports.[17-19]

Differential diagnosis of sarcoidosis and TB sometimes can be very difficult, especially in countries with high prevalence of TB. Despite the innovative diagnostic techniques, in some patients, there still persists the puzzle weather the 2 granulomatous diseases coexists, or are they followed one by another, or are they misdiagnosed.

CASE STUDIES

Case 1

In the year 1983, a patient was treated for pulmonary tuberculosis (smear positive and Lowenstein cultures positive). At that time, he was also dismissed from the military service because of *M. tuberculosis* infection (Figure 30-1).

In the year 1993, he experienced symptoms of breathlessness, weight loss, and fatigue. This time a diagnosis of pulmonary sarcoidosis was made on the basis of a positive skin biopsy. He was treated with steroid therapy. His symptoms

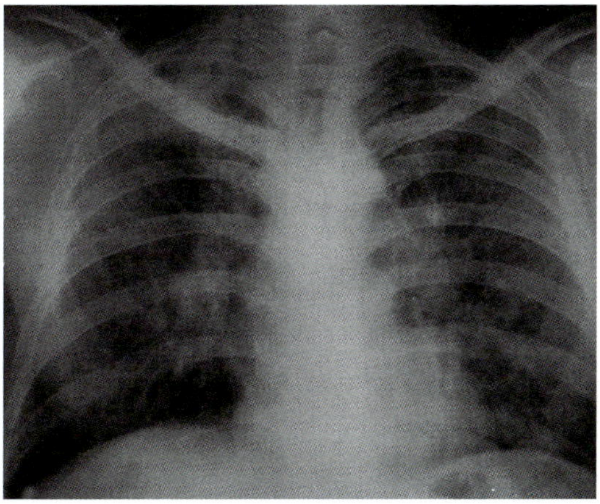

Figure 30-1 Lesions in the upper lobe of the right lung presenting tuberculosis. However, mediastinal shadow is quite suggestive of enlarged lymph nodes. In primary tuberculosis (and our patient was at the age of about 20 years while in a military service), parenchymal lesions are always accompanied by enlarged regional lymph nodes.

remitted. In the year 2000, a chest X-ray showed stage III of lung sarcoidosis (Figure 30-2). Serum angiotensin converting enzymes level was 136 U/l. Because of the previous history of TB, it was decided to perform bronchoscopy. Again, the diagnosis of pulmonary sarcoidosis (relapsing disease) was made on a positive biopsy.

Ophthalmologic examination revealed ocular sarcoidosis. Steroid therapy improved the symptoms, however, he had definite lung function impairments with decrease vital capacity (VC); diffusing capacity (DLCO) was decreased too.

In this patient, sarcoidosis followed 10 years after cured *M. tuberculosis* infection.

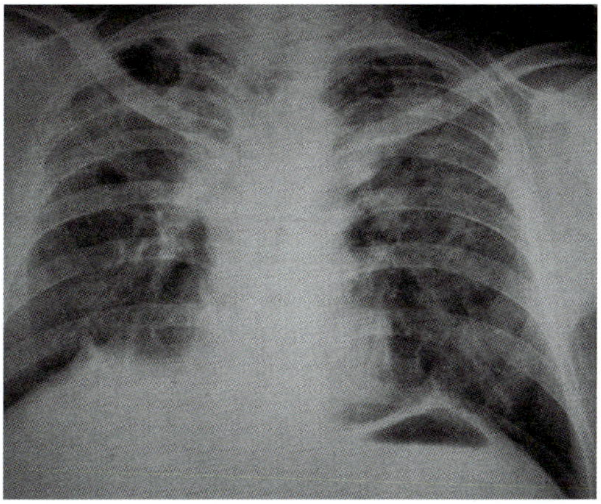

Figure 30-2 Chest X-ray presenting stage III of the lung sarcoidosis: hilar retraction, with diffuse parenchymal lesions.

CASE 2

A 64-year-old male patient was diagnosed with diabetes mellitus in 1982. Ten years later, a diagnosis of pulmonary sarcoidosis was made on a positive biopsy (1992). At that time he was on oral antidiabetic therapy. The steroid treatment was started.

In October 2002, he experienced episodes of dry hacking cough and chest discomfort. The mediastinal shadow was enlarged as presented in figure 30-4. Bronchoscopy was performed and a diagnosis of relapsing pulmonary sarcoidosis was established. At that time his serum angiotensin converting enzyme level was within normal range 39 U/L and Ca level in the urine was 7.41 mmol/L per 24 hours. Again, the steroid treatment was started due to relapse of sarcoidosis. The control X-ray (Figure 30-3) showed improvement.

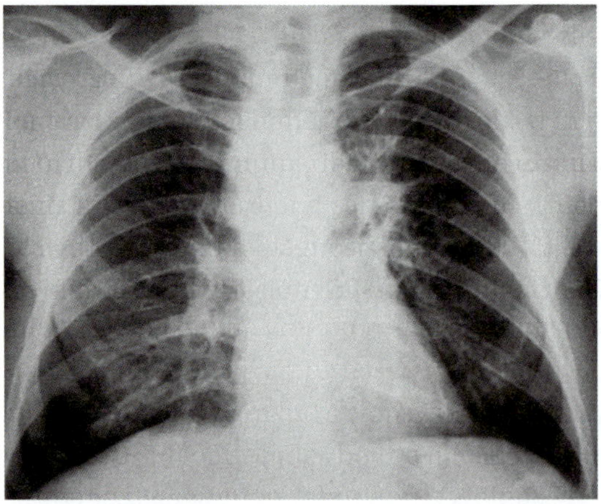

Figure 30-3 Remission of the enlarged mediastinal lymph nodes after steroid therapy.

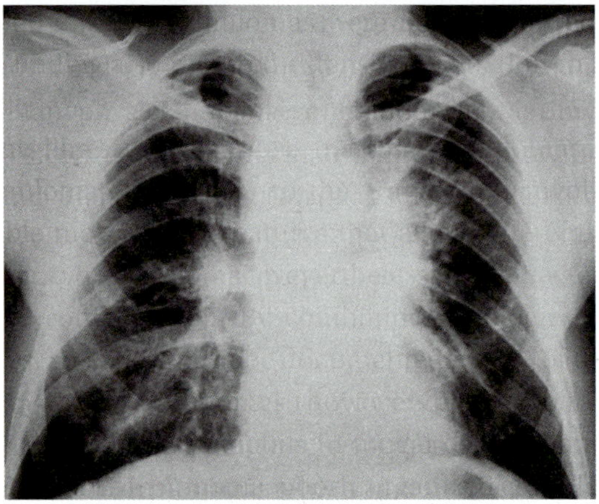

Figure 30-4 Enlarged mediastinum.

A year later in October 2003, he was admitted to the hospital emergency department because of severe dyspnea as a result of pleural effusion (Figure 30-5). Pleural biopsy revealed sarcoidosis (Figure 30-6). After steroid therapy was introduced, symptoms remission was accompanied with chest X-ray improvement (Figure 30-7).

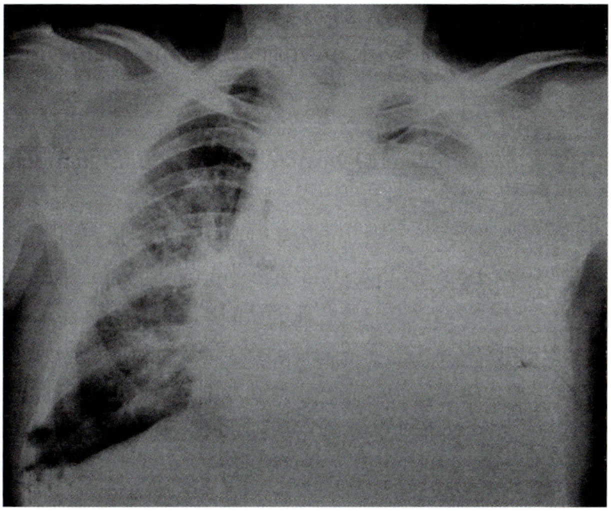

Figure 30-5 Chest X-ray presenting pleural effusion in this sarcoidosis patient.

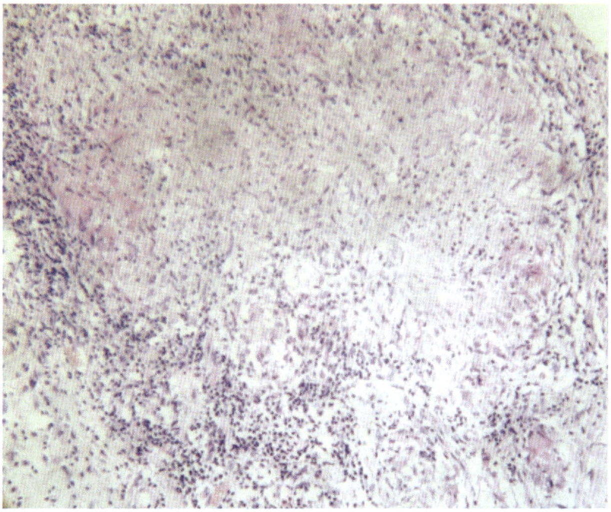

Figure 30-6 Sarcoidosis of the pleura. *Courtesy:* Dr Jelena Stojsic, MD. Service of Pathohistology, Department of Pathology, Clinic of Pulmonary Diseases and Clinic of Thoracic Surgery, Clinical Center, Belgrade, Serbia.

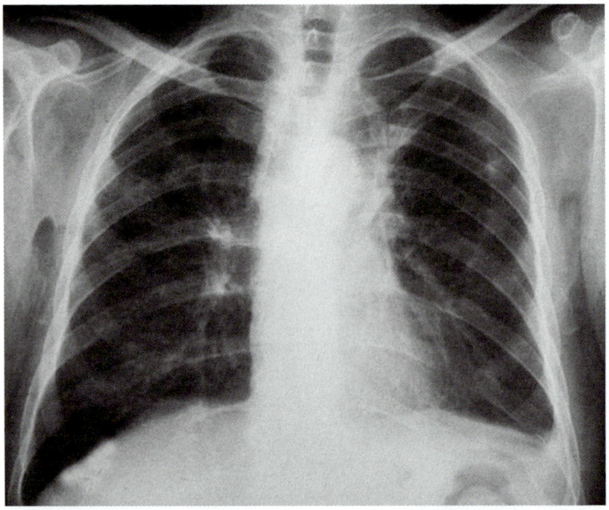

Figure 30-7 Chest X-ray representing remission of pleural sarcoidosis on steroid therapy.

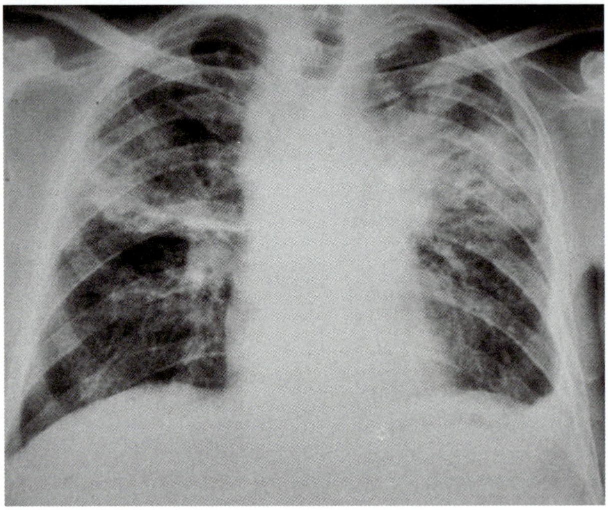

Figure 30-8 Chest X-ray revealed progression of the parenchymal lesions both lungs, this time not due to sarcoidosis.

In February 2004, he was again admitted in the hospital with dominant symptoms of cough and weight loss from time to time fever in the afternoons. Shortly after the therapy with antituberculotics was introduced, the chest X-ray improved (Figure 30-8).

The patient was smear positive, and 6 weeks later was also Lowenstein cultures positive (innumerous number of colonies).

In this patient, TB followed after sarcoidosis was treated with steroid therapy (Figure 30-9). These two cases of TB before and after sarcoidosis represents the persisting puzzle of the relationship between the two granulomatous diseases.

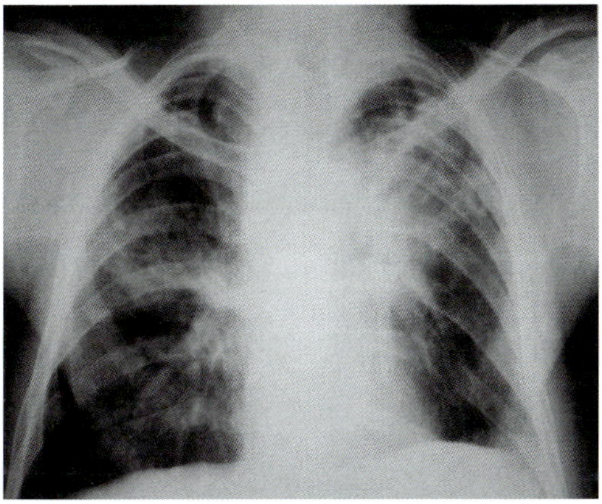

Figure 30-9 Chest X-ray of the same patient one month later, presenting improvement.

REFERENCES

1. Newman LS, Rose CS, Maier LA. Sarcoidosis. *N Engl J Med.* 1997;336:1224-33.
2. Noppen M. Tuberculosis and sarcoidosis. *Chest.* 1999;115:1480.
3. Mangiapan G, Hance AJ. Mycobacteria and sarcoidosis: an overview and summary of recent molecular data. *Sarcoidosis.* 1995;12:20-37.
4. Brett GZ. Epidemiological trends in tuberculosis and sarcoidosis in a district of London between 1958 and 1963. *Tubercle.* 1965;46:413-6.
5. Israel HL, Sones M. Sarcoidosis, tuberculosis, and tuberculin anergy: a prospective study. *Am Rev Respir Dis.* 1966;94:887-95.
6. Zaki MH, Addrizzo JR, Patton JM, et al. Further exploratory studies in sarcoidosis: an epidemiologic investigation to compare the prevalence of tuberculosis infection and/or disease among contacts of matched sarcoidosis and asthmatic patients. *Am Rev Respir Dis.* 1971;103:539-45.
7. Popper HH, Klemen H, Hoefler G, Winter E. Presence of mycobacterium DNA in sarcoidosis. *Hum Pathol.* 1997;28:796-800.
8. Inderlied CB. Mycobacteria. In: Armstrong D, Cohen J, editors. Infectious diseases. London: Mosby; 1999. p. 20-22.
9. Bocart D, Lecossier D, De Lassence A, Valeyre D, Battesti JP, Hance AJ. A search for mycobacterial DNA in granulomatous tissues from patients with sarcoidosis using the polymerase chain reaction. *Am Rev Respir Dis.* 1992;145:1142-48.
10. Schluger NW, Kinney D, Harkin TJ, Rom WN. Clinical utility of the polymerase chain reaction in diagnosis of infections due to Mycobacterium tuberculosis. *Chest.* 1994;105:1116-21.
11. Querol JM, Farga MA, Granda M, Gimeno C, Garcia-de-Lomas J. The utility of polymerase chain reaction (PCR) in the diagnosis of pulmonary tuberculosis. *Chest.* 1995;107:1631-5.

12. Bemer-Melchior P, Germaud P, Drugeon HB. Diagnosis of extrapulmonary tuberculosis by a commercial polymerase chain reaction kit. *Pathol Biol (Paris).* 1998;46:597-603.
13. Inui N, Suda T, Chida K. Use of the QUANTIFERON-TB Gold test in Japanese patients with sarcoidosis. *Respir Med.* 2008;102:313-5.
14. Golding IM, Lester W, Berg GS. Adrenocortical steroids and tuberculosis. *N Engl J Med.* 1956;254:1026-8.
15. Smyllie HC, Connolly CK. Incidence of serious complications of corticosteroid therapy in respiratory disease. *Thorax.* 1968;23:571-81.
16. Cowie RL, King LM. Pulmonary tuberculosis in corticosteroid-treated asthmatics. *S Afr Med J.* 1987;72:849-51.
17. Wong CF, Yew WW, Wong PC, Lee J. A case of concomitant tuberculosis and sarcoidosis with mycobacterial DNA present in the sarcoid lesion. *Chest.* 1998;114:626-9.
18. Knox AJ, Wardman AG, Page RL. Tuberculous pleural effusion occurring during corticosteroid treatment of sarcoidosis. *Thorax.* 1986;41:651.
19. Mise K, Goic-Barisic I, Puizina-Ivic N, Barisic I, Tonkic M, Peric I. A rare case of pulmonary tuberculosis with simultaneous pulmonary and skin sarcoidosis: a case report. *Cases J.* 2010;3:24.

CHAPTER

31 Sarcoidosis in Childhood

INCIDENCE

Sarcoidosis is a worldwide disease which occurs most often in young adults in the third and fourth decades of life.[1]

Sarcoidosis is less common in children than in adults;[2-6] that is the reason why little is known about the true incidence and prevalence, for the same reason little is known about the clinical course of sarcoidosis in children, although quite a few studies from the literature have elucidated most of the clinical presentation of the disease in children (Figure 31-1).[7]

In infants and children younger than 4 years, sarcoidosis is manifested with triad of skin, joint, and eye involvement without typical pulmonary disease.[5,8,9] Older children have typical clinical presentation of sarcoidosis with the involvement of the lungs, lymph nodes, and eyes.[10-11]

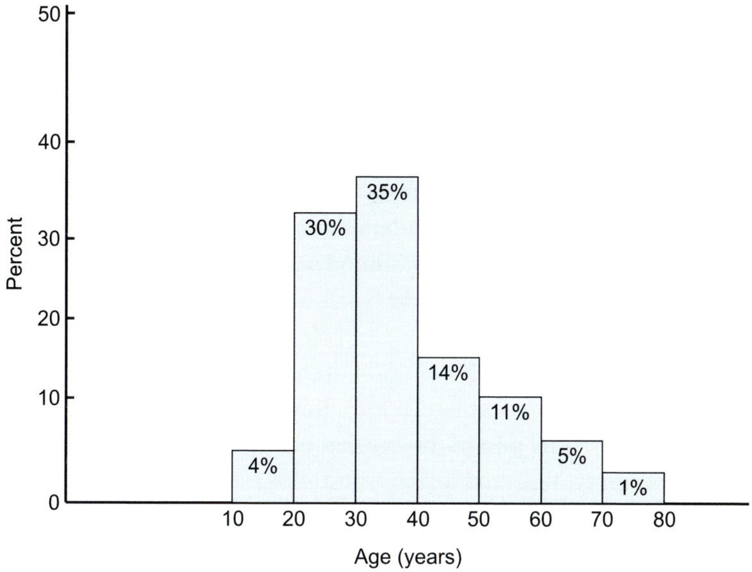

Figure 31-1 Sarcoidosis is more frequent in third and fourth decades of life. *Source:* Sharma OP. Sarcoidosis: Clinical Management. London: Butterworths; 1984. p. 5.

Majority of cases of sarcoidosis in children have been reported to occur in patients between 13-15 years of age,[2,12] however, the disease has also been reported in very young children.[7,8,13]

HISTORY

Possibly the first article on this topic was published in 1937 by Bertli Roos in Z Kinderheilkd.[14]

DIAGNOSIS

The diagnosis of sarcoidosis in childhood is established as in adult patients when a compatible clinical and radiographic picture is supported by histological evidence of noncaseating granulomas in the affected organs and exclusion of other granulomatous disease with similar histologic or clinical picture.[15,16]

Angiotensin converting enzyme (ACE) in childhood sarcoidosis is not a reliable parameter as in adults when elevated. Children, especially adolescents have significantly higher ACE. The enzyme is age and sex dependent, higher in boys, probably related to a steroid hormonal regulation of ACE synthesis. This must be taken into account for diagnosing sarcoidosis in children, following the course of the disease, and evaluating therapy effectiveness.[17]

Early onset of sarcoidosis: in children in the first 4 years of life, sarcoidosis is a rare disease, characterized by the triad of skin rash, uveitis, and arthritis.[4,8] However, pulmonary involvement is unusual in early onset of sarcoidosis but is the leading feature of late onset disease.

Clinical history and detailed physical examination should guide the physician to choose the biopsy site that can be reached in the minimal invasive way.

CLINICAL FEATURES

Majority of cases of sarcoidosis in children are accompanied by constitution symptoms like fever, fatigue and malaise, and weight loss. Older children usually present with a multisystem disease similar to adult manifestation.

Most common clinical feature in childhood sarcoidosis is peripheral lymph node enlargement.[2] Up to 70% of children with sarcoidosis have peripheral lymph nodes enlargement.[2,4,8,18,19]

Sarcoidosis of eyes is extremely common in children. In young children, it should be mandatory to perform complete ophthalmologic evaluation including split-lamp examination.[2,4,8,9] Any part of the eye can be affected in childhood sarcoidosis but the most frequently observed lesion is anterior uveitis (iritis or iridocyclitis) in approximately 58% of children with very early onset of sarcoidosis.[8,9,12] In older children, frequency of ocular disease varies between 24 and 54%.[4,8,12] Posterior segment of the eye is less commonly involved with sarcoidosis in children than in adults.

Skin involvement occurs in 24–40% of older children[4,8,12] and in 77% of very young children with sarcoidosis.[8] Erythema nodosum and Lofgren's syndrome as the hallmark of acute sarcoidosis and lupus pernio the traditional manifestation of chronic skin lesion in older women are rare in children,[16] but when present, indicate good prognosis.

Parotid gland enlargement is a frequent finding in children with sarcoidosis.[9] Heertfort's syndrome (a combination of fever, parotid gland enlargement, anterior uveitis, and cranial nerve palsies) has been reported in childhood sarcoidosis.[4,8,10]

Rare Manifestations of Childhood Sarcoidosis

Bone involvement is rare in children. Osteolytic bone lesions are rarely seen in association with musculoskeletal manifestations. Musculoskeletal features of sarcoidosis include joint effusions. Arthritis in childhood sarcoidosis can be easily confused with juvenile rheumatoid arthritis (JRA), particularly in preschool children.

Renal disease, if manifested, includes disorders of calcium homeostasis including hypercalcemia and hypercalciuria in up to 30% of children.[2] Sarcoidosis of the heart and hematologic abnormalities are rare in children.[9,16]

Baumann and Robertson, in 2003, reviewed the available literature, finding 29 case reports of childhood neurosarcoidosis. They pointed out that the symptoms differ substantially from neurosarcoidosis in adults. Prepubertal children are likely to present with seizures. The adult pattern of cranial nerve involvement appears only after puberty. Evidence of hypothalamic dysfunction is also common in children with patients showing growth failure, diabetes insipidus, and lack of sexual maturation.[18]

THERAPY

Oral steroids are indicated as the first line therapy in patients with pronounced systemic disease. Dose and duration, like in adults, must be individualized. Gedalia et al.[19] described the experience of 6 months low dose methotrexate in 7 children with biopsy-positive sarcoidosis. Methotrexate therapy resulted in improvement of clinical symptom score and decreased mean daily steroid dose.

PROGNOSIS

Sarcoidosis of childhood is a rare disease and follow-up studies describing the prognosis and natural history are lacking. Early onset of sarcoidosis with involvement of eyes, joints, and skin suggests a safeguarded prognosis with the likelihood of chronic progressive course.[7] In a recent Danish study by Milman and Hoffmman on childhood sarcoidosis, prognosis was not related to the age at onset of disease. Erythema nodosum was associated with a good prognosis and central nervous system involvement with a poor prognosis.[7]

Long-lasting clinical follow-up of every single child with sarcoidosis focusing on disease severity remains the best approach to these patients and the best way to determine the prognosis.

REFERENCES

1. Crystal RG. Sarcoidosis. In: Isselbacher K J, Braunwald E, Wilson JD, Martin JB, Fauci AS, Kasper DL, editors. Harrison's principles of internal medicine. New York: McGraw-Hill; 1994. p. 1679-84.
2. Patishall EN, Strope GL, Spinola SM, Denny FW. Childhood sarcoidosis. *J Pediatr.* 1986;108:169-77.
3. Kendig EL. Sarcoidosis. *Am J Dis Child.* 1982;136:11-2.
4. Hetherington S. Sarcoidosis in children. *Compr Ther.* 1982;8:63-8.
5. Lindsley CB, Godfrey WA. Childhood sarcoidosis manifesting as juvenile rheumatoid arthritis. *Pediatrics.* 1985;76:765-8.
6. Hoffmann AL, Milman N, Byg KE. Childhood sarcoidosis in Denmark 1979–1994: incidence, clinical features and laboratory results at presentation in 48 children. *Acta Paediatr.* 2004;93:30-6.
7. Milman N, Hoffmann AL. Childhood sarcoidosis: long-term follow-up. *Eur Respir J.* 2008;31:592-8.
8. Hetherington S. Sarcoidosis in young children. *Am J Dis Child.* 1982;136:13-5.
9. Hafner R, Vogel R. Sarcoidosis of early onset. A challenge for the pediatric rheumatologist. *Clin Exp Rheumatol.* 1993;11:685-91.
10. Patishall EN, Kendig EL. Sarcoidosis in children. *Pediatr Pulmonol.* 1996;22:195-203.
11. Shetty AK, Gedalia A. Sarcoidosis: a pediatric perspective. *Clin Pediatr.* 1998;37:707-18.
12. Kendig EL Jr. Sarcoidosis in children. Personal observations on age distribution. *Pediatric Pulmonol.* 1989;6:69-70.
13. Byg KE, Milman N, Hansen S. Sarcoidosis in Denmark 1980–1994. A registry-based incidence study comprising 5536 patients. *Sarcoidosis Vasc Diffuse Lung Dis.* 2003; 20:46-52.
14. Roos B. Uher das Vorkonnan des Schaunnanschen benignen Lymphogranulomatose (des Boeckschen genignen Milarlupoids) bei Kindern [English translation: On the incidence of Schaumann's benign lymphogranulomatosis (Boek's benign milary lupoid) in children]. *Z Kinderheilkd.* 1937;59:280-302.
15. Yammamoto M, Sharma OP, Hosoda Y. The 1991 descriptive definition of sarcoidosis. *Sarcoidosis.* 1993;9:33-4.
16. Statement on sarcoidosis. *Am J Respir Crit Care Med.* 1999;160:736-55.
17. Bénéteau-Burnat B, Baudin B, Morgant G, Baumann FC, Giboudeau J. Serum angiotensin-converting enzyme in healthy and sarcoidotic children: comparison with the reference interval for adults. *Clin Chem.* 1990;36:344-6.
18. Baumann RJ, Robertson WC Jr. Neurosarcoid presents differently in children than in adults. *Pediatrics.* 2003;112;e480-6.
19. Gedalia A, Molina JF, Ellis GS Jr, Galen W, Moore C, Espinoza LR. Methotrexate in the treatment of childhood sarcoidosis. *J Pediatr.* 1997;130:25-9.

CHAPTER

32 Sarcoidosis in the Aged

INTRODUCTION

Although sarcoidosis is considered a disease of young and middle aged adults, there have been a certain number of cases among elderly.[1] It was not always certain whether sarcoidosis in these cases was recurrence of prior disease or it represented the initial onset in old age. In a study of 115 patients with sarcoidosis, 11 (9%) were 60 years of age or older at the time of presentation. The most common symptoms were related to the respiratory system (dyspnea, cough, and chest pain), occurring in about two-thirds of all patients.[2] Remission is less likely to be achieved in elderly patients, particularly in those with extensive skin and bone involvement. However, early diagnosis and the initiation of effective therapy avert the complications of the disease.

CLINICAL PRESENTATION

Miyoshi et al. reported an interesting case of a 77-year-old Japanese male with fatigue, polydipsia, and polyuria. Central diabetes insipidus was diagnosed by depletion of vasopressin secretion in response to increases in serum osmolality. Secretory responses of anterior pituitary hormones including adrenocorticotropin, thyrotropin, gonadotropins, and growth hormone were impaired. Diffuse swelling of the infundibulum as well as lack of T1-hyperintense signal in the posterior lobe was noted by pituitary magnetic resonance imaging. Chest X-ray showed bilateral hilar lymphadenopathy and bronchoalveolar lavage fluid (BAL) demonstrated increased CD4/CD8, ratio consistent with the diagnosis of sarcoidosis. The patient was treated with corticosteroids, thyroid hormone, and desmopressin supplementation. Complete regression of the neurohypophysial swelling was notable 2 years after corticosteroid replacement.[3]

Kodama et al. reported a case of a 74-year-old woman whose symptoms of dementia may have been caused by sarcoidosis and in whom steroid treatment was effective. The patient had bilateral mediastinal adenopathy, bilateral uveitis, negative tuberculin, high serum angiotensin converting enzyme (ACE) value, and a positive Gallium-67 scan. Lymph node biopsy revealed typical granulomas compatible with

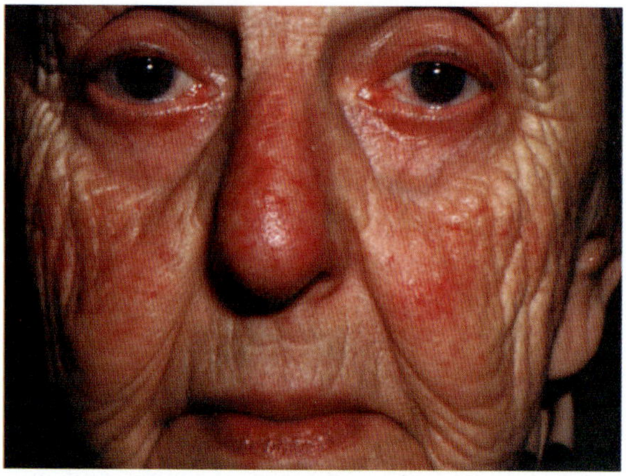

Figure 32-1 This lady was 83 years at the time she experienced relapsing sarcoidosis. For the first time, the diagnosis of sarcoidosis (with bilateral hilar adenopathy) was established on mediastinoscopy at the time she was 30. More than 50 years after that, her disease relapsed.

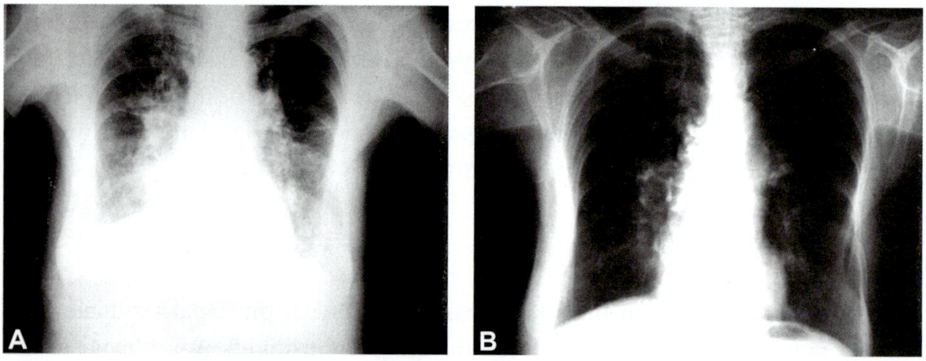

Figure 32-2 **A**, Before, and **B**, after the therapy.

sarcoidosis. The progression of dementia was shown by declining scores of mini-mental state examination (MMSE) from 17/30 on admission to 7/30 on day 30 after admission. Prednisolone (50 mg/day) was given. One month after the start of steroid treatment, the MMSE score increased to 20/30.[4]

A case report of an 83-year-old lady has been described in figure 32-1. At this time she had lupus pernio lesions on her face (Figure 32-1), fibrotic stage III of the lung sarcoidosis (Figure 32-2A), and restrictive lung function impairment. She complained of breathlessness. Fortunately, she responded nicely to steroid treatment (Figure 32-2B).

Another interesting case was of a 65-year-old man with sarcoidosis, who noticed an enlarging painless nodule in his forearm. Magnetic resonance imaging of the nodule showed a star-shaped area of lower signal intensity, surrounded by an area of higher signal intensity. Histological examination showed noncaseating granulomas.

Sarcoidosis was diagnosed. The nodule enlarged in size over a period of 8 months. Prednisone was given. Forty days later, his symptoms disappeared and the nodule dramatically shrunk.[5]

In one of our patients, a 77-year-old woman developed bilateral hilar and mediastinal lymphadenopathy (BHL) and uveitis. BHL was not present in a chest radiograph taken 6 months prior to the admission. Serum ACE was elevated, tuberculin skin test was negative, and BAL had increased number of lymphocytes (33.2%). It was clear that in this case of sarcoidosis had an elderly onset.

In the management of sarcoidosis in the aged, it is important to remember that a malignant disease of the lung, stomach, intestine, and even uterus may give rise to a granulomatous reaction in the draining lymph nodes. This local sarcoid reaction must not be confused with the multisystem sarcoidosis. Where there is a granulomatous reaction in the elderly, doubt the diagnosis of sarcoidosis, "think of neoplasia" is a helpful dictum to follow.[6]

REFERENCES

1. Spagnolo P, Luppi F, Roversi P, Cerri S, Fabbri LM, Richeldi L Sarcoidosis: challenging diagnostic aspects of an old disease. *Am J Med.* 2012 Feb;125:118-25.
2. Sharma O. Sarcoidosis in the aged. *Geriatrics* 1973;76: 50-55
3. Miyoshi T, Otsuka F, Takeda M, Inagaki K, Otani H, Ogura T, Ichiki K, Amano T, Makino H. An elderly patient with sarcoidosis manifesting panhypopituitarism with central diabetes insipidus. *Endocr J.* 2007;54:425-30. Epub 2007 Apr 20
4. Kodama M, Umegaki H, Mogi N, Iguchi A, Takeda A. An elderly case with sarcoidosis whose symptom of dementia was effectively treated by steroid. *Nihon Ronen Igakkai Zasshi.* 2002;39:648-53.
5. Aono J, Hamada H, Yokoyama A, Kondo K, Kohno N, Hiwada K.A case of sarcoidosis with muscle nodules. *Nihon Ronen Igakkai Zasshi.* 2001;38:689-92.
6. Tachibana T, Iwai K, Takemura T. Sarcoidosis in the aged: review and management. *Curr Opin Pulm Med.* 2010;16:465-71.

Index

Page numbers followed by *f* refer to figure and *t* refer to table

C

D

E

F

G

H

I

J

K

L

M

N

O

P

Q

R

S

T

U

V

W